THE TYPE 1 DIABETES COOKBOOK

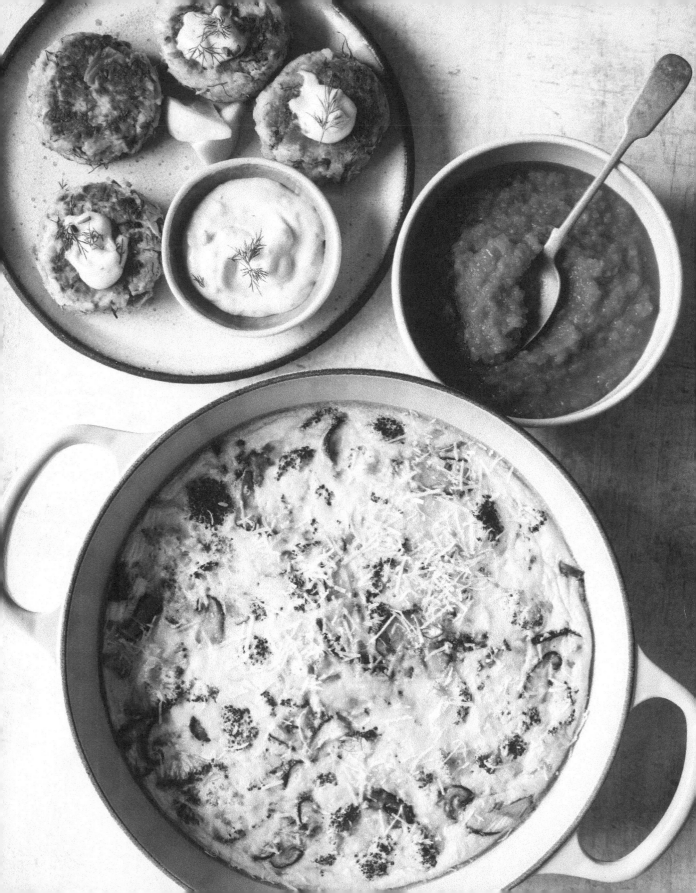

THE
TYPE 1 DIABETES
COOKBOOK

Easy Recipes for Balanced Meals
and Healthy Living

Laurie Block, MS, RDN, CDE

PHOTOGRAPHY BY NADINE GREEFF

ROCKRIDGE
PRESS

"An education is the one thing that no one can take from you."
Thank you Mom and Dad, Susie, and Uncle Norman.

Designer: Katy Brown
Editor: Meg Ilasco
Production Editor: Erum Khan
Photography © Nadine Greeff, 2018
Author photo © Donald Carlton

ISBN: Print 978-1-64152-233-5
ebook 978-1-64152-234-2

R1

Contents

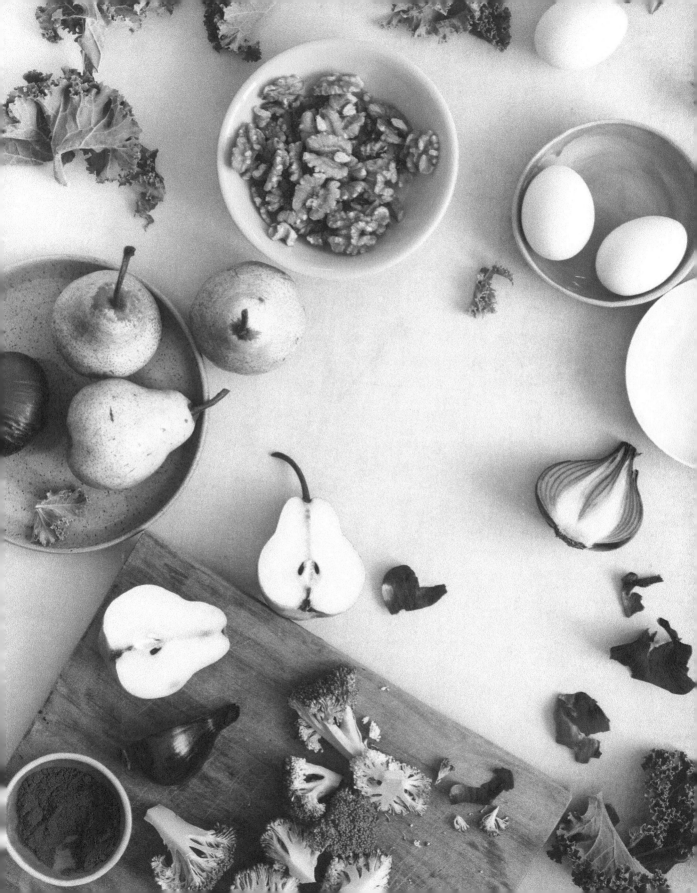

Introduction

A healthy diet really matters. I have known this since I was quite young. My family struggled with many diet-related difficulties, including diabetes, weight management issues, and heart disease. It was not a surprise that my high school yearbook quoted me as stating, "I want to become a nutritionist." That was 30 years ago, long before nutrition was front-page news. I was always interested in science and was fortunate to know what I wanted to study. I applied to the few dietetic/nutrition programs available at the time and earned my undergraduate degree in nutrition at Hunter College. Hunter College was in New York City, a city filled with culture and diversity. Students shared and ate all types of food, and the environment continued to spark my interest in foods and how different food preferences affect health.

During my internship at Mount Sinai Medical Center in 1985, physicians were studying diet as it related to diabetes. I quickly learned the differences between type 1 and type 2 diabetes. In those days, type 2 was referred to as "non-insulin-dependent diabetes," and type 1 was called "juvenile diabetes" or "insulin-dependent diabetes." The names did not make much sense, because some folks with type 2 required insulin, and not everyone with type 1 was a child!

The newly diagnosed type 1 population needed a nutrition education, quickly! They of course required insulin for survival, but they also needed information about how food and mealtimes coordinated with the action of insulin. The emphasis at the time was on meal timing, limiting simple sugars, understanding carbohydrate digestion, and creating a balanced diet.

In the 1980s, people with diabetes were taught techniques for self-monitoring of blood glucose using portable blood glucose meters that were large and cumbersome. Typically, it would take five minutes for one reading, but at least the information was available, and it was quite valuable. Individuals were able to test before and after meals, and they could really begin to understand the effects of different foods on their body. As a nutritionist, I had hard-core data: Clearly, diet really did matter!

I then enrolled in a program at New York University Steinhardt School of Culture, Education, and Human Development, and received my master's degree of science in nutrition in 1985. I wrote my thesis on diet and diabetes. Soon thereafter, I became a registered dietitian (RD) and certified diabetes educator (CDE).

With my clinical work behind me, I went on to earn a master's certificate in cooking from The New School for Social Research. Since that time, I have worked as a passionate diabetes and nutrition educator with pediatric, adolescent, and adult populations.

In the years since, I have met thousands of people living with diabetes. I've consulted family members and volunteered throughout the diabetes community. I have been, and continue to be, involved in walks, advocacy movements, and support efforts in the emotional roller coaster that comes with a diagnosis of type 1.

As an RD and a CDE, I share private and personal moments with individuals, helping them through the life-changing diagnosis and 24/7 care that diabetes requires. I now witness firsthand the power of food and what a change in diet can do for blood sugar management. I collaborate with endocrinologists and diabetes teams in hospitals, clinics, community outreach programs, and corporations. One of our goals is to translate the ever-changing science of nutrition and diabetes into actionable strategies. Ultimately, my aim is to make it easier for those living with diabetes to enjoy stability and good health, and a big part of that is reinforcing that diet really does matter!

The Type 1 Diabetes Cookbook is here to help you understand the many variables that are so important as you manage diabetes. Section by section, you'll learn about planning healthy meals, recipe substitutions, low-carbohydrate diets, glycemic load and index, the impact of cooking and food processing, how to treat low blood sugars, the value of reading nutrition labels, the myths, the truth about misleading claims, the importance of different vitamins, and how to shop wisely and establish a well-balanced diet.

Together we'll explore insulin and delivery systems, expected target goals for blood sugars, devices for self-monitoring blood glucose, insulin sensitivity/correction factors, and the newest technologies.

A section on type 1 diabetes as it pertains to the different stages of child development will help you know what to expect and help you develop strategies to ensure success at any stage of childhood.

My selection of Resources for Diabetes Education (page 144) includes links to information on lifestyle management, evidence-based studies, support groups, and community functions. It can be worthwhile to connect with others who are dealing with similar issues through online support groups and sharing ideas within the type 1 community.

And then, of course, there are the recipes! Have fun mixing and matching these recipes according to how much carbohydrate intake you are planning at meals. These recipes are moderate in carbohydrates, limit simple sugar, aim at including fiber, and include healthy fat and protein. These principles will help keep premeal and post-meal blood sugars within target ranges and support overall good health.

I know how much diet matters, so I'm delighted to share this information with you!

I

THE TYPE 1 DIABETES DIET

This book is more than just a cookbook. It's a resource to help you understand and take control of your type 1 diabetes with information, tips, tricks, and then, of course, lots of delicious recipes. This section will provide you with helpful guidance on insulin, blood glucose monitoring, pumps, and sensors. We'll also talk about how food choices can make all the difference in the management of blood sugar levels. Whether you know a lot about type 1 or are totally new to the issue, there is so much to learn, and this book is designed to help. This education will be a powerful tool and can help you build confidence so you can worry less about managing your blood sugars and spend more time enjoying life!

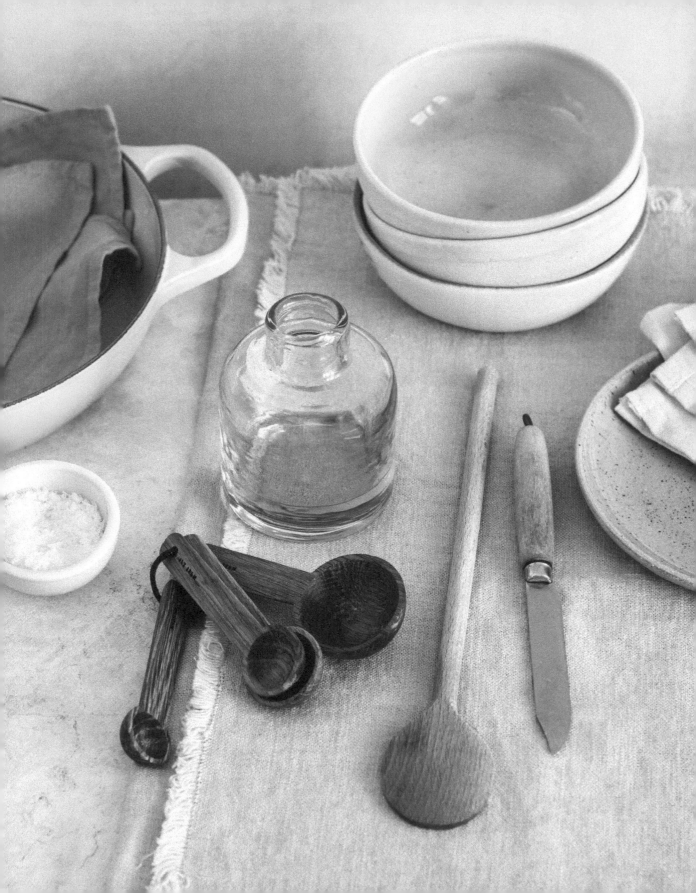

CHAPTER ONE

Getting to Know Type 1 Diabetes

Type 1 diabetes (T1D) occurs when the body is unable to produce insulin, a hormone produced by the pancreas. Although the exact cause is unknown, it is believed to be a combination of genetics and environment. Today, an estimated 1.25 million people live with T1D in the United States, and 40,000 people are diagnosed every year. T1D results when the body's immune system attacks and destroys its own cells; in this case, it kills the healthy insulin-producing cells. Without insulin from these cells, the body is unable to help sugar (glucose) enter the cells to provide energy.

In this chapter, you will learn the basics of T1D and how it differs from type 2 diabetes (T2D). We will explore the various treatments and tools for monitoring T1D, and you'll learn how these, along with dietary interventions and exercise, are key components of a plan that will help you consistently meet your target blood sugars. There are so many strategies available to make living with type 1 easier, so let's get started.

A Lifelong Condition

I wish there were another answer, but currently, management of T1D always requires insulin. Regardless of any changes you implement in your diet, vitamin intake, or lifestyle, if you are diagnosed with T1D, you will need insulin.

Insulin is an amazing hormone produced by the pancreas. The pancreas works to regulate blood sugar, or glucose, levels. It works like this: You eat something, your body digests the foods you eat, and some of that food (mostly carbohydrates but also protein and some fats) converts to glucose, which is the body's primary source of energy. Once glucose is released into the bloodstream, the pancreas responds and releases insulin, which helps move the glucose into our cells for energy. With type 1 diabetes, an outside source of insulin needs to be delivered to do the job; this is typically achieved by injecting insulin or by using an insulin pump.

T1D differs from T2D in that in type 2, the body actually produces insulin, but often the insulin that is produced does not work effectively. With T2D, oral medication, non-insulin injectables, and lifestyle changes are the primary treatments.

Understanding Insulin

When we eat foods, they get digested, carbohydrates and protein get turned to glucose, and then we need insulin to transport it from the bloodstream to the cells for energy. It's simple to comprehend, but the process is actually a complex balancing act, involving other hormones and organs (such as the liver, which stores glucose), various forms of glucose, and the process through which we derive glucose from foods. In any case, when glucose enters the bloodstream, the pancreas is responsible for responding and releasing insulin, to help bring the glucose into the cell to provide energy. As you now know, T1D requires delivery of insulin from outside the body.

There are many different types of insulin and delivery systems, and your primary health care provider can help you determine which is best for you and your lifestyle. Your initial dose will be calculated by your body weight and is called your total daily dose. Part of the total daily dose will be used to cover for your baseline needs (basal insulin), and some will be used to account for the food you are eating (bolus insulin).

PRIMARY TYPES OF INSULIN AND SCHEDULES

Rapid- or short-acting insulin: These quick-acting insulins begin their clinical effect in 5 to 30 minutes. Referred to also as bolus insulin, this variety of insulin is taken before meals to cover for food or to correct elevated blood sugars.

Long- or intermediate-acting insulin: This variety of insulin is usually taken once or twice a day and has a duration of action anywhere from 12 to 42 hours. Often referred to as basal insulin, this type of insulin works around the clock to cover for hormones and baseline needs; however, it is not used to cover for food.

Premixed insulin: This variety mixes both shorter-acting and longer-acting insulin. Premixed insulins are usually recommended for twice-daily administration and include meal coverage and baseline needs.

SLIDING-SCALE INSULIN

Some people with T1D may be provided with a "sliding scale" of insulin. Sliding-scale regimens are preset insulin doses based on premeal blood sugar readings. If your blood sugars are, for example, between 100 and 150 mg/dl before a meal, your doctor may say to take 1 unit of insulin; and if blood sugars are between 200 and 250 mg/dl, to take 2 units of insulin. Sliding scales are easy to use and do not require much math. They are preset by your health care team and adjusted as you develop blood sugar patterns. They are based only on blood sugars before meals and do not account for varying amounts of carbohydrates at meals. This insulin regimen works best if there are consistent meal schedules and carbohydrates throughout the day.

MULTIPLE-DOSE INJECTIONS

If you are not on a sliding scale, your doctor may recommend a regimen known as multiple-dose injections (MDI). Here the doctor will use a formula to calculate your insulin needs. This formula will provide you with insulin to cover for baseline needs, and an additional formula will help you understand how much insulin you will need to cover for food or to correct high blood sugars. The MDI regimen is a bit more sophisticated than others, and you will need either some math skills or a good calculator. There are basically two equations used to determine MDI formulas: the correction factor (CF) and the insulin to carb ratio.

The insulin to carb ratio is used at mealtime. The formula estimates how many units of insulin will cover for a given amount of carbohydrates. For example, if your doctor says you have an insulin to carb ratio of 1:10, this means that for every

10 grams of carbohydrates you consume, you will need 1 unit of insulin. Based on that formula, if you are eating 40 grams of carbs, you would need 4 units of insulin.

The correction factor does not consider food but rather is focused on correcting any blood sugars that are elevated out of your expected range. For example, if your premeal blood sugars are targeted to be 80 to 120 mg/dl and your actual premeal blood sugars are 300, your physician may direct you to correct them before you eat. For example, if your correction is 1:50, this means that 1 unit of insulin will lower your blood sugars 50 points. With that formula, if you give yourself 4 units of insulin, your blood sugars will lower by 200 points to 100 mg/dl.

The routine for an MDI regimen is as follows: First, test your premeal blood sugars to determine if you need correction insulin. Next, look at the food you are eating and the carbohydrate content at that meal, and then use your insulin to carb ratio to account for the carbohydrates in the meal. Yes, so much math! However, a calculator can be a tremendous help, and if you use an insulin pump, the numbers are already plugged into the pump.

Insulin Delivery Methods

Years ago, the only option available was to deliver insulin with a syringe. Today, there are many options that are quick and easy and leave less room for error.

SYRINGES

Syringes are the old-time method of delivering insulin. This method requires drawing up the insulin from a bottle into a syringe and then injecting the insulin into the tissue in different parts of your body. This requires good vision and dexterity, as you need to be accurate in drawing the correct amount of insulin into the syringe.

INSULIN PENS

An insulin pen really looks like a pen, and it is very easy to use. Some come prefilled and are completely disposable; others are reusable, and you simply change the prefilled insulin cartridge. With both styles, a very fine needle attaches to the pen that delivers insulin. There are even safety caps that go on top of the pen that can help conceal the needle. The primary advantage to insulin pens is their "dial and dose" technology. Simply dial the number of insulin units prescribed, and with a few clicks, a number appears on the pen indicating the dosage prepared. Pens are sanitary and particularly helpful for those with poor vision or dexterity issues.

INSULIN PUMPS

There are a few different types of pumps on the market. Some look like a small, cool digital gadget, cell phone, or computer mouse. Each pump contains a cartridge of insulin and delivers insulin either wirelessly or through a tube-like system. Insulin pumps come with an infusion set that has an insertion device. The insertion device has a small, fine needle that places a tiny cannula (plastic tube) just under the skin. The pump then delivers insulin through this plastic tube. Insulin pumps are pre-programmed to deliver insulin 24 hours a day. This continuous delivery of insulin is known as the basal dose and covers for baseline needs.

Basal insulin does not account for food—bolus insulin does that job. The bolus feature on the pump has two main functions: to account for food and to correct for elevated blood sugars. The bolus calculator is used to account for the carbohydrate component in an upcoming meal or snack. By entering the amount of carbohydrates you are eating, the pump will be preprogrammed to deliver the necessary amount of bolus insulin. The correction bolus is used to deliver insulin to correct blood sugars that are outside of the recommended range before a meal or at other times of the day.

The basal and bolus features on the pump work together to stabilize blood sugars without multiple daily injections. Other advantages of insulin pumps include precise and flexible insulin delivery. Insulin pumps still require some effort—you will need to enter blood glucose readings, have an understanding of the carbohydrate component of meals, and change insertion sites. Before starting with an insulin pump, it's important to understand the basics of insulin injections and carbohydrate counting.

INHALED INSULIN

Wow, wait! No needles? Yes, there is a rapid-acting insulin that is inhaled and absorbed through the lungs. This form of insulin can be used at mealtimes and snack times to cover for the carbohydrates you are eating. However, inhaled insulin does not provide the very important background insulin coverage required for baseline needs in type 1 diabetes. It has recently been approved only for adults with type 1 and type 2 diabetes, with contraindications for anyone who has lung disease. You may want to ask your health care team if inhaled insulin is right for you.

Monitoring Blood Glucose

Blood sugar or blood glucose monitoring lets you know what your blood sugars are at any given moment. There are all sorts of devices on the market. Traditional meters are simple to read and provide valuable information. A newer technology is the continuous glucose monitoring (CGM) system. This system uses a sensor to read glucose levels and has the ability to display individual readings on receivers or smartphones.

GLUCOSE METERS

Blood glucose meters are easy to use. These small and portable devices come with disposable test strips that you insert into the machine. All you need is a tiny drop of blood from the finger to dab on the strip, and in just five seconds, you get a blood sugar reading. These meters come with a lancing device that uses a penlet (looks like a pen) and a lancet (a tiny needle). Fingerstick blood testing is easy, relatively painless (especially if you prick the side of your finger), and quick, providing immediate blood sugar results anywhere you are.

CONTINUOUS GLUCOSE MONITORING

If you want to reduce the frequency of fingersticks associated with traditional glucose meters, you may wish to ask your diabetes team about CGM, or continuous glucose monitoring. This technology uses a device that inserts a sensor under the skin to measure glucose. Every five minutes, the sensor reads blood sugars and sends the reading to an app on your smartphone or receiver, which displays the readings continuously. Some sensors are worn on the back of your arm and you wave a receiver over the sensor to tell you your readings. Other sensors wirelessly transmit glucose readings to certain insulin pumps and actually communicate with the pump to help determine how much background insulin you need. Without numerous fingersticks, you will be able to get as many as 288 blood glucose readings per day. This technology allows you to see if your blood sugars are trending high or low and to share your readings with family members or others in your support system. Sensors have all kinds of helpful features, including graphs showing blood sugar trends, and can alert you if blood sugars run high or low. The graphs will also help your health care team fine-tune your insulin doses. Sensors do not eliminate fingersticks altogether; sometimes it's necessary to double-check things or calibrate the sensor.

What Should Your Blood Sugars Be?

People who do not have diabetes normally have very stable blood sugars in the range of 70 to 120 mg/dl throughout the entire day. For those with diabetes, the goal ranges from 80 to 180 mg/dl, accounting for pre- and post-meal readings. The ranges are a bit more liberalized but are consistent with an important study called the Diabetes Control and Complication Trial. This study concluded that blood sugars that are near normal and are controlled with intensive insulin therapy result in less frequent diabetes-related complications. (Your endocrinologist or diabetes doctor will discuss this with your individualized goals.) It is important to remember that these are ranges and that many factors, such as pregnancy, age, and living situation, influence target goals.

The American Diabetes Association's 2018 Standards of Care comprised the following target goals for people with T1D; however, other organizations believe that blood sugar targets should be more in line with the levels of people who do not have diabetes.

BEFORE MEALS (PRANDIAL)

Target level: 80 to 130 mg/dl

Premeal testing shows how accurately you dosed for a previous meal or if baseline insulin needs to be adjusted. Results will be high if you used too little insulin to cover for a previous meal or snack. Many factors unrelated to food can contribute to high or low blood sugars before meals.

AFTER MEALS (POSTPRANDIAL)

Target level: Less than 180 mg/dl (varies by individual)

Postprandial testing will determine how well your insulin dose is controlling your blood sugars about one to two hours after a meal. If the number is too high, you may need a slightly larger dose, and if it is too low, you may want to lower your dose. Post-meal blood sugar testing accounts for the glucose effects of certain foods, the composition of your meals, the amount of fiber, and whether lifestyle or exercise routines have changed.

HEMOGLOBIN A1C (HBA1C) BLOOD TEST

Target level for adults: Less than 7 percent
Target level for children: Less than 7.5 percent
Target level for some seniors* and infants: Less than 8 percent

This blood test shows the average blood sugars over a two- to three-month period. This test is most frequently done in the doctor's office two to four times per year, and blood is typically drawn from the arm. You can ask if your health care team does point-of-care testing, which gives you results of the A1C test with just a prick of the finger, similar to the fingerstick used in self-monitoring for blood glucose.

* Some seniors live alone, and as such, it is preferable that they keep their blood sugar levels a bit higher, to prevent issues related to low blood sugars.

Testing Blood Glucose

You can keep blood sugars steady with all the tools available to you, including your medication, glucose meters, and sensors. Enlist your support systems, including the health care team, family, and friends, to help. Maintaining steady blood sugars requires a fine balancing act, and the more you understand about your condition and how your body responds to all the various factors, the greater success you will experience. How and when you monitor blood glucose is highly individualized. In general, consider the following guidelines for when to check it:

- As requested by your health care team

- Before meals to determine how much insulin you will need based on the amount of carbs you are eating and to see if you need to correct elevated blood sugars

- Again about 90 minutes after eating to determine if your insulin-to-carbohydrate ratio needs adjustment

- More frequently when you are not feeling well

- Before and after exercise or if activity routines change

- If you have symptoms or suspect low blood sugars

- Anytime you want information on how your blood sugars are trending (consider a continuous glucose monitor)

TREATING HIGH OR LOW BLOOD SUGARS

We know that maintaining steady blood sugar levels is important. However, even with consistent routines, healthy eating, and regular exercise, blood sugars can still rise or fall to levels that require attention.

HYPOGLYCEMIA

Hypoglycemia, or low blood sugars, occurs when blood sugars fall under 70 mg/dl. If your blood sugars are trending low, speak with your doctor about adjusting your insulin. If low blood sugars occur only on occasion, try the 15/15 rule: Consume 15 grams of simple carbohydrates, such as juice, hard candy, or glucose tablets; wait 15 minutes; and test blood sugars. Repeat this process until blood sugars have risen. Eating protein after treating low blood sugars can be helpful in stabilizing sugar levels. If your blood sugars are so low that you cannot eat or drink, try putting glucose gels or honey on the inside of your cheek or under your tongue. For severe hypoglycemia, ask your health care team about an emergency injectable hormone called glucagon. Glucagon acts within 15 minutes and directs your liver to release stored glucose into the bloodstream. If you are unconscious or unable to swallow, your support system can confirm low blood sugars with a fingerstick, administer glucagon, and call 911. Be sure to discuss signs of low blood sugars with loved ones and teach them to administer glucagon so they can help you if needed. Some signs and symptoms of low blood sugars include confusion, nervousness, slurring words, shaking, sweating, headaches, and numbness in the arms and legs. Wear medical identification, which can prove invaluable if you need assistance with low blood sugars.

HYPERGLYCEMIA

Hyperglycemia, or high blood sugars, is defined as levels above 126 mg/dl; however, treatment definition varies between individuals. Often, high blood sugars can result from inadequate insulin, excessive carbohydrates, illness, hormones, or stress. You may have symptoms such as thirst or increased urination as your body attempts to get rid of the sugars in the bloodstream. It is likely that insulin adjustment will be necessary, although sometimes it's just about remembering to take your insulin!

Your doctor may ask you to test your urine for ketones if your blood sugar is greater than 250 mg/dl. Ketones are acids that develop when the body attempts to break down fat or protein for energy. This occurs when there is not enough glucose in the cells. Without enough insulin, sugars will remain in the blood, and the cells will not get the glucose they need. The cells will then turn to other sources, such as protein or fat, for energy. However, fats and protein do not provide glucose and instead will form acids, which change the acidity of your blood. This condition, referred to as DKA, or ketoacidosis, is life-threatening. The failure to take insulin is the number-one cause of ketoacidosis. Speak to your doctor about getting ketone strips to test your urine when blood sugars are elevated or especially during illness. It is also important to stay hydrated when blood sugars are elevated.

The Role of a Healthy Diet

There is no exact diabetes diet—even nutritionists and diabetes educators debate the recommendations. However, there are common principles that we do understand about food and nutrition and how they relate to blood sugar levels and overall health. Our diets generally have three main nutrients that are important for growth and development and to help stabilize blood sugars and provide energy: carbohydrates, protein, and fats. All have different effects on blood sugars, but they are each important for a balanced diet.

MACRONUTRIENTS, VITAMINS, AND MINERALS

Macronutrients are nutrients that are needed in relatively large amounts. These include carbohydrates, protein, and fats. While many diets encourage people to eliminate carbs or fats, I believe it is best to avoid fad diets that eliminate or severely limit a whole category of foods.

Carbohydrates are plentiful in most people's diets. Carbs are primarily found in grains and flours, fruits, milk and dairy, vegetables, beans, and simple sugars, such as honey and sugar. Carbohydrates are also found in alternative sugars, such as sorbitol or mannitol. Everyone needs carbs to maintain energy, receive necessary fiber for healthy digestion, and supply the body with vitamins and minerals. Carbs are also the key component that creates insulin demand. How much carbohydrate intake one needs remains under debate among health professionals. Most would agree the quality of carbs is important. Limit simple sugars and carbodydrates with excess sodium, and choose high-fiber grains.

Protein is found in meats, poultry, eggs, cheese, fish and seafood, and plant sources such as tofu, nuts and nut butters, and beans. Protein is necessary for many important functions, such as building and repairing tissue, as well as maintaining lean muscle mass. Most people with diabetes don't realize that large quantities of protein have the ability to raise blood sugar levels. It's just a longer and less efficient process; typically glucose rises 4 to 12 hours after a high-protein meal. Individuals respond very differently to protein in their diet. A general guideline to account for protein is to consider 6 to 7 ounces a moderate portion. For each additional 3 ounces of protein, count the protein as if you were consuming 20 grams of carbohydrates. Check your blood sugars, consider a CGM device, and speak with your team about how you can divide insulin doses or adjust pump settings with protein meals.

Remember to consider amounts of protein not only for blood sugars, but also if you notice any weight gain.

Fats are found primarily in butter, oils, nuts, avocados, cheeses, and fatty meats. We need fat to help the body absorb fat-soluble vitamins as well as to provide energy, support healthy skin and hair, and enable cell growth. Like protein, fats do not turn immediately to glucose, and they have little effect on blood sugars. However, fats do play a role in how fast carbohydrates are digested and can cause delayed hyperglycemia. Fats also tend to be high in calories. Just 1 teaspoon of oil or butter contains 45 calories, and foods like nuts and salad dressings are also relatively high in calories. With that in mind, if you are gaining weight and relying on foods high in fat because they "don't require insulin," you may want to consider how much fat you are eating.

Calcium is found in milk, leafy greens, fortified cereals, tofu, almonds, and dairy products. This important mineral plays a role in blood pressure, muscle contractions, hormone secretions, and of course, bone health. For individuals with type 1 diabetes, getting enough calcium in combination with vitamin D is important for development of strong bones and teeth and to maintain structure. The National Institutes of Health recommends 200 to 260 mg calcium daily from 0 to 12 months; 700 milligrams daily between the ages of 1 and 3; 1000 mg between ages 4 and 8; 1300 milligrams between ages 9 and 18; 1000 milligrams between ages 19 and 70; and 1200 milligrams for those over age 70. Discuss the need for calcium supplements if you are avoiding dairy products or food sources of calcium.

Vitamin D is found in fatty fish, such as salmon, trout, swordfish, and sardines, and fortified milk products. Another way to get vitamin D is to expose the legs or arms (without sunscreen) to the ultraviolet B rays of the sun for 5 to 15 minutes daily, two to three times per week. This will activate the natural process that produces vitamin D. Vitamin D and calcium work together and are essential for bone growth and prevention of osteoporosis. Recent research provides evidence that vitamin D may improve immune function, increase insulin sensitivity, and help with overall glucose control. Additional studies demonstrate that individuals with low levels of vitamin D may be more prone to develop type 1 diabetes. Your health team will check your levels and determine if a supplement is necessary. Many organizations, such as the Vitamin D Council and the Endocrine Society, recommend higher doses than the National Institutes of Health (NIH). The NIH recommends the following for each age-group: infants 0 to 12 months, 400 IU daily; ages 1 to 70, 600 IU daily; and ages over 70, 800 IU daily.

Carbohydrate Counting

Carbohydrates are the primary macronutrient responsible for raising blood sugars. All of the carbohydrates you eat get digested within one to two hours. Quick-acting sugars, like juice, may act in five minutes, whereas more complex starches, such as bread, raise blood sugars more slowly. Whichever carbohydrate you choose, it's important to understand that the total carbohydrate intake at each meal should be coordinated with insulin action.

Counting carbohydrates is quite easy. Many resources list the carbohydrate content of the foods you eat (see Resources for Diabetes Education, page 144). Take advantage of nutrition labels on food products and carb-counting applications on your smartphone (many are listed on page 144) so you can begin to gain a better understanding of carbohydrate counts in the various food groups.

The first step to counting carbs requires understanding which foods contain carbohydrates and what equals a serving size. Measuring cups and/or a digital food

WHAT ABOUT LOW-CARB DIETS?

Low-carbohydrate diets, such as Atkins, Protein Power, or the ketogenic diet, are making headline news and are extremely controversial. There is evidence that low-carb diets may help with weight reduction, and there are long-standing studies that show limiting carbohydrates can prevent seizures in individuals with epilepsy. However, there is not sufficient evidence to warrant low-carbohydrate diets for all patients with type 1 diabetes. Low-carb diets may translate to lower insulin dosing, but this does not necessarily mean that such diets are beneficial to overall health. Before recommending or advocating any extreme diets, I look at the entire medical history, check kidney function, cholesterol levels, and blood sugars, and then discuss how much carbohydrate

intake is indicated for that individual. The Academy of Nutrition and Dietetics does not have any specific guidelines for carbohydrate intake; however, according to the National Academy of Medicine, the minimum requirement is 130 grams daily. Recommendations by many health organizations indicate carbohydrates at each meal. A typical distribution looks like this: 30 to 45 grams carbohydrates at breakfast; 5 to 25 grams at snacks; 30 to 60 grams at lunch, and 30 to 60 grams at dinner. Athletes may need much higher carbohydrate intake. Keep an open mind and look at new evidence-based publications to understand how low-carb diets with less than 50 grams of carbs daily fit into the world of type 1 diabetes and the ever-changing science of nutrition.

scale will prove handy tools in your kitchen. All nutrition labels list the serving in ounces or weight in grams, so you'll want a scale that has both ounces and grams. The following chart provides general information about carbohydrate values in different food groups. Appendix C (page 140) also lists carbohydrate counts of various diverse foods.

Protein and fats do not contain significant amounts of carbohydrates and are not traditionally accounted for when carbohydrate counting. If you eat large quantities of fat or protein, you may need to consider this when calculating your insulin dose. Refer to "How Many Carbohydrates Do You Need?" (page 139) for an estimate based on your estimated energy intake.

CARBOHYDRATE CONTENT IN FOOD GROUPS

FOOD GROUP	CARBOHYDRATE GRAMS	EXAMPLE
Starch	15	1-ounce slice whole-wheat bread
		⅓ cup rice or pasta
		½ cup beans
		½ English muffin
		¾ cup cold cereal
		½ cup peas or corn
		1 cup butternut squash
Fruit	15	1 small apple or 4 ounces of juice
		½ banana, mango, or pear
		15 to 17 grapes
		1¼ cups strawberries
		12 cherries
Milk	15	8 ounces milk
		8 ounces yogurt
		8 ounces soy milk
Meat and Protein	0	1 ounce chicken, fish, or turkey
		1 ounce beef or pork
		1 egg
		3 egg whites
		4 ounces tofu
Fats	0	1 teaspoon butter or oil
		1 tablespoon cream cheese
		⅛ avocado
		1 slice bacon
Vegetables	5	½ cup cooked vegetables
		½ cup corn or peas
		1 cup raw vegetables

Glycemic Index and Glycemic Load

The glycemic index (GI) is a measurement system for ranking individual foods according to the blood glucose response after meals. Foods with a low GI (55 or lower) are expected to slowly increase blood sugars, foods with a medium GI (56 to 69) indicate a more moderate rise, and foods with a high GI (over 70) may cause a rapid blood sugar response. GI charts can be helpful, but keep in mind that the GI index does not consider typical portions, fiber content, particle size, and how foods are used in the context of a meal.

The glycemic load (GL) is believed to be a more accurate tool for measuring foods by their post-meal blood glucose response. GL considers both the GI index and the quantity you are eating. To determine a food's GL, multiply the GI by the number of carbohydrate grams in a serving, and then divide by 100. A low GL is between 1 and 10; a moderate GL is 11 to 19; and a high GL is 20 or higher. You may notice some foods have a low glycemic load but a high glycemic index. This is simply because the glycemic index does not consider portions.

While both GI and GL can help you anticipate how your body may react, the best advice is to test blood sugars before and after meals and determine your individual response to foods. A well-balanced diet includes foods with a low or medium GL or GI from all food groups. Visit the University of Sydney's glycemic index, www.glycemic index.com/foodSearch.php, for detailed information on glycemic load and index.

LOW GLYCEMIC INDEX (55 OR LOWER)	MEDIUM GLYCEMIC INDEX (56 TO 69)	HIGH GLYCEMIC INDEX (70 AND GREATER)
Apple	Couscous	Corn flakes
Barley	Dates	Corn sugar (dextrose)
Corn tortilla	French fries	Instant mashed potatoes
Fruit sugar (fructose)	Ice cream	Instant oat porridge
Green banana, boiled	Pineapple	Jelly beans
Kidney beans	Popcorn	Potato, boiled
Lentils	Pumpkin, boiled	Rice crackers
Milk, skim or low fat	Quick oats	Rice milk
Peanuts	Sweetened soft drinks	Rice porridge/congee
Pumpernickel	Wheat roti	Saltine crackers
Soybeans	Whole-wheat bread	White bread
Steel-cut oatmeal	Wild rice	White rice

DIETARY FACTORS THAT INFLUENCE BLOOD SUGARS

Several factors influence how quickly carbs are absorbed. You'll want to consider the following:

Carbohydrate type: The type of carbs you eat will affect how quickly your blood sugars rise. There are two types of carbs: simple carbohydrates, which raise blood sugars very quickly and include things like sugar, white bread, white rice, and baked goods, and complex carbohydrates, which include whole grains, legumes, and vegetables. Stay focused on limiting simple carbohydrates and understanding total carbohydrate intake.

What you eat with the carbs: Eating a mixed meal with both fats and protein will affect how quickly carbohydrates are digested. Fat and protein slow down the digestion and absorption of carbohydrate foods. This explains why meals high in fat or protein may need insulin doses to be divided and why it is not recommended to rely on chocolate bars or high-fat ice cream to treat low blood sugars.

The form of the carbs: Carbs consumed as liquid (such as juice) generally have little fat or fiber, so they are absorbed quickly and potentially will raise blood sugars rapidly. Other factors, such as glycemic index, fiber content, cooking time, and even the ripeness of a fruit, can affect the impact of carbohydrates and post-meal blood sugars.

How fast you eat them: Starting a meal with simple sugars may not coordinate well with insulin action. Try eating protein first if you see that your blood sugars are elevated at the start of the meal.

Alcohol: Plan to eat something if you drink alcohol. Don't drink on an empty stomach. Alcohol can cause blood sugars to lower and cause symptoms that are similar to those of intoxication. A small snack of cheese and crackers or nuts and crackers should help prevent low blood sugars that can accompany alcohol consumption. Like anything, moderation is key to keeping blood sugars stable. The basic guideline is not to exceed one alcohol equivalent for women and two alcohol equivalents for men. One alcohol equivalent is equal to 12 ounces of beer, 4 ounces of wine, or 1½ ounces of a distilled spirit, such as vodka.

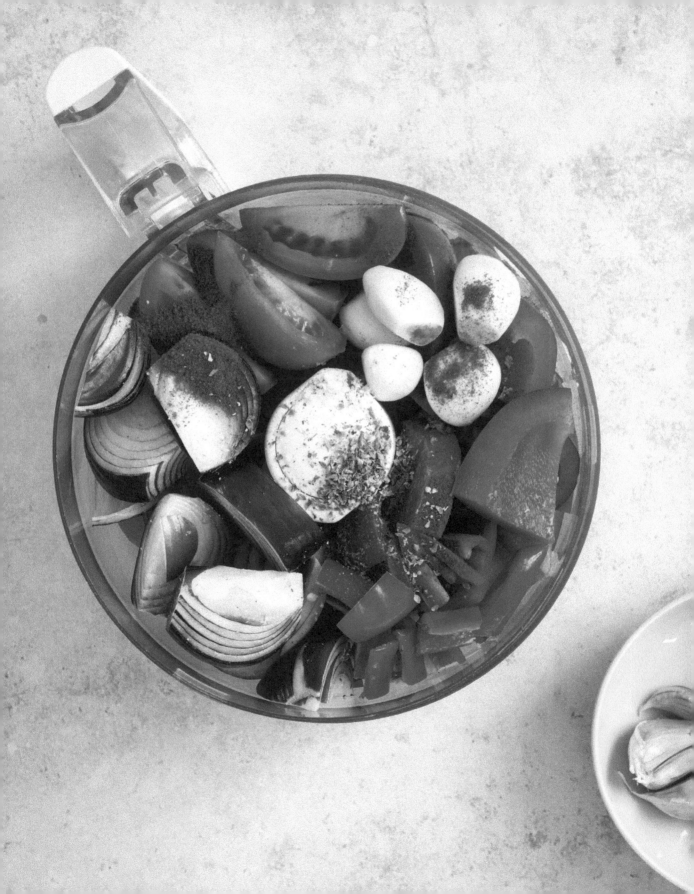

CHAPTER TWO

Preparing to Make Healthy Changes

It can seem overwhelming to make major dietary changes, particularly those that require you to do a lot of food preparation. I want to assure you that a little planning will go a long way in making these changes easier to implement. There are three things I recommend that can make your transition smoother: Plan meals for the week ahead, shop from a list, and keep your kitchen stocked with some necessary equipment and pantry items. These tricks will save you from making impulse purchases and running back out to the store to get what you need. A little planning will put you in control and make it easier to adapt to a new and healthy lifestyle.

Type 1 Diet Essentials

The following dietary guidelines will be helpful to anyone with type 1 diabetes.

Aim for a balanced diet. Seek out carbohydrates that are full of fiber, such as whole grains, fresh fruits, and nonprocessed vegetables. Include fish three times per week, as well as lean meats and calcium-rich protein sources, like tofu and milk. Use healthy fats, such as monounsaturated fat–these include olive and avocado oils, seeds, nuts, and nut butters. Enjoy caffeine and alcohol in moderation, limit simple sugars, and drink plenty of water.

Understand insulin action and meal timing. If you're unclear about how to time your insulin and meals, please discuss this with your diabetes educator. To be effective, insulin and meal timing need to coordinate; this will also help prevent low and high blood sugars.

Read labels. Reading labels is one of the most important things you can do in the grocery store. Become a label-reading pro! In doing so, try not to fall for any misleading claims, like those that read "sugar-free" or "no added sugar." Look at serving sizes and total grams of carbohydrates. Aim for products with at least 3 grams of fiber per 100 calories and less than 5 grams of sugar.

Include healthy proteins. Protein is essential for cell growth and repair. Include healthy, lean proteins, such as fish, tofu, or poultry. You will not take insulin to cover for protein portions unless you are eating unusually large amounts compared to your regular intake.

Carry a simple form of sugar. Keep portable snacks with you, like juice boxes, sports drinks, hard candy, jelly beans, dried fruit, honey, or glucose tablets or gels. You may need them to treat low blood sugars. Even with the best of intentions, low blood sugars can occur, so be prepared by keeping simple sugars on hand.

If you drink alcohol, eat when you do. Surprisingly, alcohol can lower blood sugars. It's always a good idea to eat some form of carbohydrates when you have a cocktail. Talk to your doctor about the best way to manage food, alcohol, and insulin.

Drink plenty of water. Is there any diet that doesn't advocate water? This diet is no different. In fact, it may be even more important for people with diabetes, since people with diabetes are at higher risk for dehydration. Don't wait until you're thirsty, and try to drink 8 to 10 glasses of water throughout the day. Also, limit beverages containing caffeine! Aim for less than 250 milligrams of caffeine daily.

BUILDING THE PERFECT PLATE

The key to a healthy diet is eating balanced meals. There is not really one perfect plate; however, I do like the Idaho plate method, which comprises 50 percent of the plate from non-starchy fruits and vegetables, 25 percent from healthy protein, and 25 percent from whole grains. The American Diabetes Association also has a fun interactive tool, called "Create Your Plate," that can be accessed online via diabetes.org.

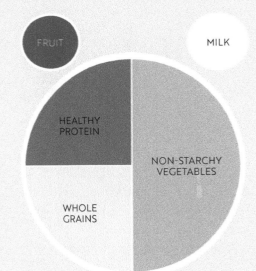

PORTIONS

It is important to understand portion size to accurately determine how much you are eating and the carbohydrate content of your meals. A good set of measuring cups, spoons, and a digital scale will be helpful to ensure the most precise measurements. If you do not have measuring tools, take a look at the following chart that provides some visual comparisons.

MEASUREMENT	COMPARISON
½ cup	Light bulb
¾ cup	Tennis ball
1 cup	Baseball
1 ounce	Ice cube or 4 small dice
3 ounces	Computer mouse
¼ cup	Egg
1 teaspoon	Fingertip
1 tablespoon	Poker chip

Adjusting for Physical Activity Levels

Exercise is important for everyone's overall health and well-being, and exercise is a great tool for lowering blood sugars. Exercise allows glucose to enter the cells more quickly and can make your body more sensitive to insulin, sometimes even lowering the amount of insulin needed. You can exercise to your heart's content; the important factor is to exercise mindfully–this may mean more frequent monitoring, glancing at your CGM device, adding a snack, or adjusting insulin doses. You don't need to be a professional to get the benefits of exercise. But there are many professional athletes living with type 1 diabetes, which illustrates how this diagnosis comes with no physical limitations. Look at the biographies of Jay Cutler, Kelli Kuehne, Sherri Turner, Lewis Marnell, Chris Dudley, Zippora Karz, Gary Hall, and Wasim Akram. Very inspirational!

The following tips are important to adjust for physical activity:

1. **Test your blood sugars right before exercise to get a baseline and to ensure you aren't starting out too low or too high.** If too low, eat something light before you start to exercise, and wait to ensure that blood sugars are rising. A typical recommendation is to eat 15 grams of carbohydrates, such as four to six crackers with an ounce of cheese. A safe range for most individuals to begin exercise is when glucose levels are between 90 and 150 mg/dl.

2. **Keep on hand some form of simple carbohydrates, such as glucose gels or tablets or raisins.** You may need simple sugars if your blood sugars are falling during or even after your exercise. Remember, exercise can have a 24-hour lowering effect on blood glucose.

3. **If you use an insulin pump, talk to your doctor about any adjustments in your pump settings.** This is especially important with strenuous exercise.

4. **"Hypoglycemia unawareness," or the inability to detect symptoms of low blood sugars, may occur during or after exercise.** Wear medical identification when exercising, and inform any exercise companions about the protocol for low blood sugars. Having glucagon on hand may be helpful, as well.

5. **Test for ketones.** If blood sugars are greater than 250 mg/dl and moderate or large ketones are present, exercise may increase blood sugar. Speak with your health care team to better understand how to exercise safely.

Adjusting in the Early Years

Adults with T1D can generally learn what to do to care for themselves. However, if you are the caregiver of a child with T1D, you'll want to know that different ages present unique challenges in managing blood sugars. Imagine, for example, all the growth spurts, varying physical activity, and appetite changes that occur during the early years. Here are some considerations to make throughout childhood.

INFANCY TO 18 MONTHS

Infants can have diabetes, and target goals are often more liberalized. The cornerstones of management are insulin and dosing off amounts of breast milk and formula. Varying appetites can make diabetes a challenge. With the introduction of solid foods, it becomes a bit easier, but close contact with your child's endocrine team and diabetes educator will be important during these earliest years.

TODDLERS AND PRESCHOOLERS

Toddlers are unpredictable, picky eaters. They tend to graze throughout the day, and (understandably) *really dislike* fingersticks and insulin syringes! Your child's doctor will likely tell you to administer insulin immediately after you know what your child eats, rather than the typical recommendation of planning insulin doses before the meal. This will allow for the unpredictability of the meal. Do not be overly concerned if your child is choosing from only one food group or has food or insulin refusal. This is quite normal, but also where discipline issues begin. You can help by modeling healthy food behaviors and introducing your toddler to healthy and nutritious foods in all sorts of colors and textures. A hands-on approach and presenting food in creative ways can also help your child learn to accept new foods. Good news—you can also consider insulin pumps or CGM systems.

SCHOOL-AGE CHILDREN AND PRETEENS

School-age children are now off and running, and you may feel a loss of parental control. The school nurse will be involved in these years and can be a wonderful ally on this journey. See if there are other children at school who have type 1, and let your child know they are not the only kid living with meters, insulin, and carbohydrate counting. You will be filling out forms for accommodations, such as a 504 Plan, to ensure your child gets the support he or she needs. School nurses can administer insulin; however, many children do not want to be called away from fun activities for nursing visits. Low-carbohydrate snacks, such as cheese sticks, pepperoni, olives, and nuts, can be helpful for blood sugar regulation if your child does not want to take an insulin dose at school. It may be easier to provide a carbohydrate snack, such as apples or crackers, when your child comes home from school, as you will then be able to provide insulin coverage.

TEENS

Teens are more concerned with peer pressure, and diabetes is not exactly their idea of fun. Often, teens will not want to do regular fingersticks, wear medical identification, or eat healthy foods. Teens may suddenly desire to change the type of insulin delivery system or detach from a pump or sensor. Issues such as fixation on body image, eating disorders, and manipulation of insulin doses result in weight loss. Teenagers who are trying to be independent may communicate less with parents or health care providers. Counseling, peer support groups, and communication with your diabetes team will be most helpful.

Smart Shopping

You don't need to spend your entire paycheck on "diabetes foods," organic foods, or specialty foods if you are living with type 1. Here are a few tips to make shopping for meals easy and effective:

Shop primarily around the edges of the grocery store. This is often where all of the most nutritious and unprocessed foods are located.

Shop with a list. Plan meals and snacks for the week ahead, before the start of each week, and write your lists from the recipes you're planning. Buy any perishable produce for the first half of the week along with any other foods you'll need, and then pop by the grocery store midweek to stock up on perishable produce you might need for the second half of the week.

Shop from home. Many supermarkets offer online shopping. You may pay a fee for the service, but you'll save in the long run when you're not tempted by unhealthy impulse items in the store.

KNOW THE DIRTY DOZEN™ AND THE CLEAN 15™

The fact that a food is organic does not change its carbohydrate count. Organic products may be free of pesticides and antibiotics, but carb values do not change. Knowing that some produce is more impacted by pesticides than others may help you choose your organics wisely. Check out the Environmental Working Group website (ewg .org) to understand which foods are part of the Clean 15™—that is, the fruits and vegetables with the smallest amount of pesticides. These are usually items with a peel, such as melons, mangos, and eggplants. You'll also see which produce is on the Dirty Dozen™, the items with the most pesticide contamination. These are the ones most worth investing your organic dollar in—often foods with thin or no skins, such as spinach, grapes, apples, and strawberries.

Reading Nutrition Labels

Nutrition labels can prove invaluable in managing your T1D. Serving size and total carbs are especially important to note. The total carbs number is the most important; in fact, look at that instead of sugars. Many people will look at sugars, and if the number is low, they believe they can eat as much as they would like. It is more important to look at total carbs, since the total carbohydrate number incorporates the amount of sugars into that number. You'll need to know this number when calculating carbs for your insulin. And don't be misled by the number of grams listed near the serving size–that measures the weight, not the carb content.

Some other things on labels that may apply to T1D include:

Sugar-free foods are not necessarily carbohydrate-free. Foods that are labeled "sugar-free" are sometimes naturally high in sugar or may contain alternative sugars, such as sugar alcohols like sorbitol or mannitol. These are carbohydrates and have potential to raise blood sugar levels.

Nutrition Facts	
8 servings per container	
Serving size	**2/3 cup (55g)**
Amount per serving	
Calories	**230**
	% Daily Value*
Total Fat 8g	**10%**
Saturated Fat 1g	**5%**
Trans Fat 0g	
Cholesterol 0mg	**0%**
Sodium 160mg	**7%**
Total Carbohydrate 37g	**13%**
Dietary Fiber 4g	**14%**
Total Sugars 12g	
Includes 10g Added Sugars	**20%**
Protein 3g	
Vitamin D 2mcg	10%
Calcium 260mg	20%
Iron 8mg	45%
Potassium 240mg	6%

* The % Daily Value (DV) tells you how much a nutrient in a serving of food contributes to a daily diet. 2,000 calories a day is used for general nutrition advice.

Net carbs are a measure of total carbohydrates minus any fiber and/or sugar alcohols (sometimes called diabetic sugars). Since there is no legal definition for net carbs, the best way to understand this measurement is to look at the total carbohydrates. If fiber or sugar alcohols are more than 5 grams, take half of the number and subtract it from the number of total carbohydrates. For example, if a product has 20 grams of total carbohydrates and 8 grams of fiber, subtract 4 (half of 8) grams from the total carbohydrates, and calculate the product as having 16 grams of carbohydrates. This will help you arrive at a more accurate count.

Gluten-free (GF) does not mean carbohydrate-free. Gluten is the general name for proteins that give elasticity to dough. You will find gluten in carbohydrate foods such as wheat, rye, and barley. Carbohydrates without gluten that earn the "gluten-free" label include rice, corn, quinoa and cassava. Other GF foods include fruit, milk, meats, fish and vegetables. Check out celiac.org to learn about GF foods and T1D. It is estimated that 10 percent of individuals with T1D also have celiac disease and need to avoid gluten. It's important to recognize that many GF foods are not carb-free and will require insulin! Read labels for carb count and monitor your response to GF foods.

Establishing Healthy Habits

Along with eating the right foods, making healthy lifestyle choices can go a long way toward helping you manage your T1D and improving your overall quality of life. While these recommendations are important for anyone, they are especially important for people with T1D because stress and unhealthy lifestyle choices may affect blood sugars.

EXERCISE REGULARLY

Exercise helps improve glucose levels and can especially help with post-meal blood sugars. You may need to make adjustments in your insulin dosage when you participate in strenuous exercise. In addition to helping with blood sugars, exercise has so many other benefits, including improving heart health and reducing stress. The recommendation for adults is a minimum of at least two hours and 30 minutes every week, plus muscle-strengthening exercise two or more days a week. Children need 60 minutes of exercise each day. Here are some tips to make exercise rewarding and successful:

HELPFUL SWAPS AND SUBSTITUTES

Try some of these simple swaps and substitutions for lower-carbohydrate versions of your favorite foods. These swaps are easy and still keep your meals quite flavorful.

Instead of noodles, make zoodles. Zucchini noodles (or noodles made from other non-starchy veggies) are a great substitute in pasta dishes. If you don't have a spiralizer, your grocery store may sell a variety of veggie noodles in the produce section. You can also make them by peeling long strips of zucchini with a vegetable peeler and then using a sharp knife to cut them lengthwise into long noodles.

Instead of rice, try cauliflower rice. It's easy to make. Grate a head of cauliflower on a box grater, and voilà! Rice! You can also pulse cauliflower florets in a food processor until they resemble rice. Once you've got your rice-size cauliflower, sauté for about 5 minutes on the stove top in a few teaspoons of oil.

Instead of potatoes, substitute another less starchy root veggie, such as turnips or celeriac. Artichoke hearts also make a nice low-carb purée to replace mashed potatoes.

When you're craving crunch, enjoy Garlic Kale Chips (page 50) instead of potato chips. You can also make yummy baked radish chips by slicing radishes thin and baking them at 375°F for 15 to 20 minutes, flipping once midway.

Instead of bread for sandwiches and wraps, use large lettuce leaves to wrap your fillings.

Instead of milk, use almond milk, which is lower in carbs and sugars than dairy milk.

Instead of white flour, use almond flour, coconut flour, or buckwheat flour.

Instead of bread crumbs, use almond meal. This works well both for coatings and as filler in meatballs and meatloaf.

Instead of ketchup, use salsa or mustard.

Instead of crackers, use Baked Parmesan Crisps (page 60).

If you like sweet tea, substitute a small amount of stevia and a squeeze of lemon for sugar.

1. **Find a type of exercise you love.** If you don't enjoy a particular exercise, it's unlikely you'll continue doing it long-term. Find something that sounds fun to you—play a sport, dance, or go for long nature walks.

2. **Preplan for exercise.** If you set aside time for exercise every day and make that important "me time," you're less likely to skip it. Pick a time of day when you are most energized and when you have had something to eat.

3. **Exercise with others.** Try planning social activities around exercise rather than around meals.

4. **Exercise with consideration to where you inject your insulin.** For example, you may want to avoid injecting insulin into the leg if you are about to go running. Injecting at the site you are about to exercise may speed up insulin absorption.

GET GOOD SLEEP

Your body needs sleep to restore itself physically, and lack of sleep can raise blood sugars. It's essential to aim for seven to eight hours of high-quality sleep per night. Here are some tips for getting good rest:

1. **Take nighttime insulin at a consistent time.**

2. **Establish a bedtime routine that gently and quietly leads you toward relaxation and sleep.**

3. **Turn off all backlit screens, including televisions, computers, and cell phones, at least an hour prior to bedtime.**

4. **If you're having trouble sleeping, try progressively relaxing each muscle group from toes to head.**

5. **Consider a white-noise generator, which may help improve sleep.**

MANAGE STRESS

Stress releases all sorts of hormones, including cortisol and adrenaline, that can make your blood sugars rise. Therefore, stress management is an important part of your overall diabetes management goals. Aim to focus on stress management three to five days per week, for about 30 minutes.

1. **Try meditation to help reduce stress levels.** Just five minutes a day of some type of meditative activity, such as focusing on breathing, can positively affect stress levels.

2. **Carve out "me time" every day.** Try to take at least 30 minutes to do something you enjoy daily.

3. **Learn to say no.** You don't always need to say yes to every request. It's okay and even cathartic to say, "That doesn't work for me right now, but thanks for thinking of me."

Vacations, Holiday Meals, and More

Planning ahead for vacation meals, holiday gatherings, and social occasions will help make living with diabetes easier. Try to forecast some of the obstacles you will face when you are eating for special occasions and are in a different environment. Here are a few tips to keep in mind that will help you sail successfully through any occasion.

EATING OUT

If you're headed to a restaurant, scope out the menu online before going, and identify a few good choices. When you arrive, ask your server how each dish is prepared. Don't be afraid to ask for simple modifications, and once the dish arrives, keep an eye on what is considered a portion. Remember the timing of your insulin and bring your supplies with you; if you are on the pump, remember to bolus insulin. Taking insulin an hour after you arrive home from a big restaurant meal often does not work to keep post-meal blood sugars in range.

SPECIAL OCCASIONS

Depending on how close you are with the host of an event, you might let that person know about your dietary preferences. If you are uncomfortable doing so, bring some of your own food to share with others. If you are going to indulge, have insulin available for the additional carbohydrates, use your carbohydrate counting skills, and enjoy your time!

VACATIONING

Planning for vacations is essential. Stock up on extra medication, supplies, pump batteries, syringes, snacks, and a glucagon emergency kit. Carry medical identification and supplies with you when you fly. Do not leave supplies in your checked luggage. Ask your health care team how to adjust insulin doses through time zones. Scope out restaurants online in advance, and plan on having a great time. There are no limits on places you can go or things you can do on vacation. A good health care team and your support system will help you manage all the way to Timbuktu and back!

About the Recipes

The recipes in this book were designed to be easy to follow. They all have 10 or fewer easy-to-find ingredients and simple step-by-step instructions. In the recipes, you'll find the following:

RECIPE LABELS

There are several recipe labels to give you more information about the recipes.

- ≤10: The recipe contains less than or equal to 10 grams of carbs per serving.

- ≤15: The recipe contains less than or equal to 15 grams of carbs per serving (but greater than 10).

- Dairy-Free: The recipe does not include dairy in the main ingredients list.

- Gluten-Free: The recipe has no gluten-containing ingredients or includes a gluten-free option.

- One-Pot: The entire meal can be prepared in one vessel (bowl, blender, skillet, baking sheet, etc.).

- Nut-Free: The recipe does not include nuts.

- Vegan/Vegetarian: The recipe is vegan or vegetarian (or includes a modification tip that makes it so).

NUTRITION INFORMATION

This includes calories and the main macronutrients. Of special importance to you are carbs (in grams per serving) and fiber. Also, if you choose to vary the recipe, you may need to recalculate the carbohydrate count using a nutrition recipe analyzer (see Resources for Diabetes Education, page 144).

II

RECIPES FOR MANAGING TYPE 1 DIABETES

Broccoli and Mushroom Frittata, page 44

Breakfast

CINNAMON OVERNIGHT OATS

GLUTEN-FREE · DAIRY-FREE · ONE POT · VEGAN

SERVES 1 · PREP TIME: 5 MINUTES, PLUS OVERNIGHT TO REFRIGERATE · COOK TIME: NONE

Overnight oats are easy to make; simply mix all the ingredients in a mason jar or single-serving container, refrigerate overnight, and they're ready to go in the morning. The whole-grain oats provide a healthy source of carbohydrates and soluble fiber, while nuts add additional protein. They come together with apples and cinnamon for a flavorful morning meal. Try variations with ¼ teaspoon of ground ginger or a pinch of freshly ground nutmeg.

⅓ cup unsweetened almond milk

⅓ cup rolled oats (use gluten-free if necessary)

¼ apple, cored and finely chopped

2 tablespoons chopped walnuts

½ teaspoon cinnamon

Pinch sea salt

PER SERVING Calories: 242; Total Fat: 12g; Saturated Fat: 1g; Sodium: 97mg; Carbohydrates: 30g; Fiber: 6g; Protein: 6g

1. In a single-serving container or mason jar, combine all of the ingredients and mix well.

2. Cover and refrigerate overnight.

STORAGE NOTE: You can make these up to 3 days ahead. You may need to adjust the liquid by adding additional almond milk after the first day. Store tightly sealed in the refrigerator.

RECIPE TIP: You can change the amount of oats or almond milk or even add a sliced apple depending upon how much carbohydrate content you desire. If you want more calories but minimal carbs, add more walnuts. Adding walnuts should not change how much insulin you need, but adding more fruit or almond milk will change the carb count.

HAM AND CHEESE ENGLISH MUFFIN MELT

NUT-FREE

SERVES 2 · PREP TIME: 10 MINUTES · COOK TIME: 5 MINUTES

A hearty breakfast sandwich doesn't need to take much time out of your morning to make. These tasty open-faced sandwiches make good use of ham and sweet tomatoes, and may contain enough carbs, protein, and fat to sustain you throughout the morning. Look for a whole-grain English muffin that contains 3 grams of fiber.

1 whole-grain English muffin, split and toasted

2 teaspoons Dijon mustard

2 slices tomato

4 thin slices deli ham

½ cup shredded Cheddar cheese

2 large eggs, fried (optional)

PER SERVING Calories: 234; Total Fat: 13g; Saturated Fat: 7g; Sodium: 834mg; Carbohydrates: 16g; Fiber: 3g; Protein: 16g

1. Preheat the oven broiler on high.

2. Spread each toasted English muffin half with 1 teaspoon of mustard, and place them on a rimmed baking sheet, cut-side up.

3. Top each with a tomato slice and 2 slices of ham. Sprinkle each with half of the cheese.

4. Broil in the preheated oven until the cheese melts, 2 to 3 minutes.

5. Serve immediately, topped with a fried egg, if desired.

STORAGE NOTE: These don't store well. Make them on demand.

RECIPE TIP: For a few more carbs, top your sandwich with another half of an English muffin, or try a dense whole-grain bread. One ounce of bread has 15 grams of carbohydrates, and you may need those extra carbs, especially if you are exercising in the morning. For fewer calories without changing the carbohydrate component, omit the ham or egg.

PUMPKIN WALNUT SMOOTHIE BOWL

≤15 · GLUTEN-FREE · ONE-POT · VEGETARIAN

SERVES 2 · PREP TIME: 5 MINUTES · COOK TIME: NONE

Here's an easy and tasty breakfast that will provide calcium and vitamin D. Smoothie bowls are thick enough to eat with a spoon. This recipe uses nutritious pumpkin purée and walnuts to provide a touch of protein and healthy omega fatty acids. Be sure to purchase pumpkin purée made only of pure pumpkin. Many people purchase pumpkin pie mix by accident, which has added sugar and spices. Remember to test blood sugars afterward to see if this healthy breakfast is matched correctly with your insulin.

1 cup plain Greek yogurt

½ cup canned pumpkin purée (not pumpkin pie mix)

1 teaspoon pumpkin pie spice

2 (1-gram) packets stevia

½ teaspoon vanilla extract

Pinch sea salt

½ cup chopped walnuts

PER SERVING Calories: 292; Total Fat: 23g; Saturated Fat: 4g; Sodium: 85mg; Carbohydrates: 15g; Fiber: 4g; Protein: 9g

1. In a bowl, whisk together the yogurt, pumpkin purée, pumpkin pie spice, stevia, vanilla, and salt (or blend in a blender).

2. Spoon into two bowls. Serve topped with the chopped walnuts.

STORAGE NOTE: You can make these the night before and refrigerate them covered overnight, but don't add the walnuts until the morning. Tightly sealed and refrigerated, these will keep for up to 3 days.

RECIPE TIP: Need a boost of carbs for a workout or low blood sugars? Add half of a chopped apple for about 8 grams of carbs. If you feel hungry after this meal, try adding more nuts the next time you make it.

AVOCADO TOAST WITH TOMATO AND COTTAGE CHEESE

NUT-FREE · ONE-POT · VEGETARIAN

SERVES 2 · PREP TIME: 5 MINUTES · COOK TIME: NONE

This creamy twist on avocado toast includes high-protein cottage cheese, which is also an excellent source of calcium, vitamin D, and heart-healthy fats. You can add up to ½ teaspoon of hot sauce if you want, depending on how much heat you want (none at all is fine, too), or you can add a dash of cayenne. Be careful—a little hot sauce goes a long way!

½ cup cottage cheese
½ avocado, mashed
1 teaspoon Dijon mustard
Dash hot sauce (optional)
2 slices whole-grain bread, toasted
2 slices tomato

PER SERVING Calories: 179; Total Fat: 8g; Saturated Fat: 2g; Sodium: 327mg; Carbohydrates: 17g; Fiber: 4g; Protein: 11g

1. In a small bowl, mix together the cottage cheese, avocado, mustard, and hot sauce, if using, until well mixed.

2. Spread the mixture on the toast.

3. Top each piece of toast with a tomato slice.

STORAGE NOTE: These need to be eaten just after they are made. Once avocado is mashed, it oxidizes quickly unless it is acidulated (has added acid, like lemon juice) and stored without any air touching its surface, so it's always best to mash avocado just before using it.

RECIPE TIP: Add 2 tablespoons of pumpkin or sunflower seeds to the cottage cheese—it brings a delightful crunch to the dish.

GINGER BLACKBERRY BLISS SMOOTHIE BOWL

≤15 · GLUTEN-FREE · ONE-POT · VEGETARIAN

SERVES 2 · PREP TIME: 5 MINUTES · COOK TIME: NONE

This low-glycemic smoothie bowl features fresh ginger, which adds a lovely flavor. You can also use fresh turmeric if you like a stronger flavor. This smoothie bowl should work to keep post-meal blood sugars in target ranges, but check blood sugars one to two hours after you eat this healthy smoothie to make sure.

½ cup frozen blackberries

1 cup plain Greek yogurt

1 cup baby spinach

½ cup unsweetened almond milk

½ teaspoon peeled and grated fresh ginger

¼ cup chopped pecans

PER SERVING Calories: 202; Total Fat: 15g; Saturated Fat: 3g; Sodium: 104mg; Carbohydrates: 15g; Fiber: 4g; Protein: 7g

1. In a blender or food processor, combine the blackberries, yogurt, spinach, almond milk, and ginger. Blend until smooth.

2. Spoon the mixture into two bowls.

3. Top each bowl with 2 tablespoons of chopped pecans and serve.

STORAGE NOTE: Since frozen berries add texture here, you can't make these ahead and store them, but they just take a few minutes in the morning to make.

RECIPE TIP: Add 2 more cups of baby spinach if you need more volume or fiber. You can also increase the amount of pecans, which will add a little extra protein, carbohydrates, and healthy fats.

HEART-HEALTHY YOGURT PARFAITS

GLUTEN-FREE · VEGETARIAN

SERVES 2 · PREP TIME: 10 MINUTES · COOK TIME: 5 MINUTES

If you want a taste of the tropics, try these tasty yogurt parfaits. Broiling the pineapple brings out its sweetness and adds caramelized flavors, and the combination of macadamia nuts, pineapple, and coconut is the perfect tropical mixture.

1 cup fresh pineapple chunks

1 cup plain Greek yogurt

¼ cup canned coconut milk

¼ cup flaxseed

2 tablespoons unsweetened toasted coconut flakes

2 tablespoons chopped macadamia nuts

STORAGE NOTE: This is best if made at the time of serving and not stored. You can mix the yogurt, coconut milk, and flaxseed and store it for up to 3 days, tightly sealed, and then broil the pineapple and assemble at a later time if you wish.

PER SERVING Calories: 402; Total Fat: 31g; Saturated Fat: 15g; Sodium: 71mg; Carbohydrates: 26g; Fiber: 9g; Protein: 10g

1. Preheat the oven broiler on high.

2. Spread the pineapple chunks in a single layer on a rimmed baking sheet.

3. Broil until the pineapple begins to brown, 4 to 5 minutes.

4. In a small bowl, whisk together the yogurt, coconut milk, and flaxseed. Spoon the mixture into two bowls. Top with the pineapple chunks.

5. Serve with the coconut flakes and chopped macadamia nuts sprinkled over the top.

RECIPE TIP: It's easy to add variety to a yogurt parfait. If you are adding fruit, be sure to consider how much that changes the carbohydrate amount. Test your blood sugars after this meal. Many people have a difficult time keeping post-meal blood sugars in check after eating fruit in the morning. If this is the case for you, add more noncarbohydrate ingredients, such as coconut flakes or slivered almonds.

LOW-CARB PEANUT BUTTER PANCAKES

≤10 · DAIRY-FREE · GLUTEN-FREE · VEGETARIAN

SERVES 2 · PREP TIME: 10 MINUTES · COOK TIME: 10 MINUTES

Pancakes don't take long to make, and you can even cook them ahead and reheat (see Storage Note) or enjoy them cold, spread with peanut butter, if you're on the go. These pancakes have a nice puffy texture from the sparkling water—you can omit it and use flat water if you don't mind flatter pancakes.

1 cup almond flour

½ teaspoon baking soda

Pinch sea salt

2 large eggs

¼ cup sparkling water (plain, unsweetened)

2 tablespoons canola oil, plus more for cooking

4 tablespoons peanut butter

STORAGE NOTE: You can make the pancakes ahead and store them in a resealable bag in the refrigerator for up to 3 days. Reheat in the toaster oven at 350°F for about 5 minutes. Spread the peanut butter over the top just before serving.

PER SERVING Calories: 454; Total Fat: 41g; Saturated Fat: 6g; Sodium: 408mg; Carbohydrates: 8g; Fiber: 3g; Protein: 17g

1. Heat a nonstick griddle over medium-high heat.

2. In a small bowl, whisk together the almond flour, baking soda, and salt.

3. In a glass measuring cup, whisk together the eggs, water, and oil.

4. Pour the liquid ingredients into the dry ingredients, and mix gently until just combined.

5. Brush a small amount of canola oil onto the griddle.

6. Using all of the batter, spoon four pancakes onto the griddle.

7. Cook until set on one side, about 3 minutes. Flip with a spatula and continue cooking on the other side.

8. Before serving, spread each pancake with 1 tablespoon of the peanut butter.

RECIPE TIP: For additional carbohydrates, add up to ½ cup of blueberries (5 grams of carbs per ¼ cup), sprinkling the blueberries over the uncooked top of the pancakes as the first side cooks, and then flip to finish cooking.

TOADS IN HOLES

≤15 · NUT-FREE · ONE-POT · VEGETARIAN

SERVES 2 · PREP TIME: 5 MINUTES · COOK TIME: 5 MINUTES

Kids and adults alike love this fun and easy breakfast with a great name. Once you crack into that semicooked egg yolk and it runs all over the bread, it's very satisfying and delicious. You can add a dash of hot sauce after it's cooked for additional flavor and serve it alongside a sliced avocado (see Recipe Tip).

2 tablespoons butter

2 slices whole-wheat bread

2 large eggs

Sea salt

Freshly ground black pepper

STORAGE NOTE: This is another one you can't make ahead, but it is fast—about 5 minutes from start to finish.

PER SERVING Calories: 241; Total Fat: 17g; Saturated Fat: 9g; Sodium: 307mg; Carbohydrates: 12g; Fiber: 2g; Protein: 10g

1. In a medium nonstick skillet over medium heat, heat the butter until it bubbles.

2. As the butter heats, cut a 3-inch hole in the middle of each piece of bread. Discard the centers.

3. Place the bread pieces in the butter in the pan. Carefully crack an egg into the hole of each piece of bread.

4. Cook until the bread crisps and the egg whites set, about 3 minutes.

5. Flip and cook just until the yolk is almost set, 1 to 2 minutes more.

6. Season to taste with the salt and pepper.

RECIPE TIP: Adding sliced avocado (either on top or on the side) is a great way to add some healthy fat and a very small amount of carbohydrates. Try mashing your avocado with 1 teaspoon of fresh lime juice and 1 tablespoon of finely chopped red onion for a quick guacamole to spread, so it becomes toads-in-holes avocado toast.

VEGGIE AND EGG WHITE SCRAMBLE WITH PEPPER JACK CHEESE

≤10 · GLUTEN-FREE · NUT-FREE · VEGETARIAN

SERVES 2 · PREP TIME: 5 MINUTES · COOK TIME: 10 MINUTES

If your doctor has told you to lower your cholesterol, you can make an egg white scramble. If not, feel free to use whole eggs. With pepper Jack cheese, onions, and green bell peppers, this is a great alternative to *huevos rancheros*, adding vibrant Southwestern flavors.

2 tablespoons extra-virgin olive oil

½ red onion, finely chopped

1 green bell pepper, seeded and finely chopped

8 large egg whites (or 4 whole large eggs), beaten

½ teaspoon sea salt

2 ounces grated pepper Jack cheese

Salsa (optional, for serving)

STORAGE NOTE: Eggs aren't great reheated, but they're passable. You can make this ahead and store it, tightly sealed in the refrigerator, for up to 3 days.

PER SERVING Calories: 314; Total Fat: 23g; Saturated Fat: 8g; Sodium: 977mg; Carbohydrates: 6g; Fiber: 1g; Protein: 22g

1. In a medium nonstick skillet over medium-high heat, heat the olive oil until it shimmers.

2. Add the onion and bell pepper and cook, stirring occasionally, until the vegetables begin to brown, about 5 minutes.

3. Meanwhile, in a small bowl, whisk together the egg whites and salt.

4. Add the egg whites to the pan and cook, stirring, until the whites set, about 3 minutes. Add the cheese. Cook, stirring, 1 minute more.

5. Serve topped with salsa, if desired.

RECIPE TIP: Add up to ¼ cup of drained and rinsed canned black beans when you add the eggs. Beans have a low glycemic index, and ¼ cup of beans has an estimated 10 grams of carbohydrates. They are an excellent source of protein, iron, and soluble fiber.

TOFU, KALE, AND MUSHROOM BREAKFAST SCRAMBLE

≤15 · GLUTEN-FREE · DAIRY-FREE · NUT-FREE · ONE-POT · VEGAN

SERVES 2 · PREP TIME: 5 MINUTES · COOK TIME: 10 MINUTES

Who needs eggs for breakfast? Get a healthy dose of vegan protein and delicious, nutritious veggies with this simple scramble. The garlic, onions, and red pepper flakes add subtle heat and spice to boost the flavor, and the tofu and mushrooms are a good source of fiber and macronutrients. If you want eggs in place of the tofu, omit the tofu and whisk together 4 eggs. Add them after the garlic, red pepper flakes, and salt, and scramble for a couple of minutes.

2 tablespoons extra-virgin olive oil

½ red onion, finely chopped

8 ounces mushrooms, sliced

1 cup chopped kale

8 ounces tofu, cut into pieces

2 garlic cloves, minced

Pinch red pepper flakes

½ teaspoon sea salt

⅛ teaspoon freshly ground black pepper

STORAGE NOTE: You can make this ahead and reheat it in the microwave or on the stove top. Store it for up to 3 days, tightly sealed, in the refrigerator.

PER SERVING Calories: 234; Total Fat: 16g; Saturated Fat: 2g; Sodium: 673mg; Carbohydrates: 12g; Fiber: 2g; Protein: 13g

1. In a medium nonstick skillet over medium-high heat, heat the olive oil until it shimmers.

2. Add the onion, mushrooms, and kale. Cook, stirring occasionally, until the vegetables begin to brown, about 5 minutes.

3. Add the tofu. Cook, stirring, until the tofu starts to brown, 3 to 4 minutes more.

4. Add the garlic, red pepper flakes, salt, and pepper. Cook, stirring constantly, for 30 seconds more.

RECIPE TIP: You may want to add some carbohydrates to this high-protein breakfast. Whole-grain toast, pita bread, and English muffins with fiber could all be good choices. Just look at the nutrition label for total carbohydrates, and aim for grains with 3 grams of fiber per 100 calories.

BROCCOLI AND MUSHROOM FRITTATA

≤10 · DAIRY-FREE · GLUTEN-FREE · NUT-FREE · VEGETARIAN

SERVES 4 · PREP TIME: 5 MINUTES · COOK TIME: 10 MINUTES

This recipe calls for shiitake mushrooms, which have a meaty texture and a hearty flavor. If you can't find them, go ahead and just use sliced button mushrooms. The flavor and texture are slightly different, but still delicious. You can also use broccolini in place of the broccoli for a slightly milder flavor.

2 tablespoons extra-virgin olive oil

½ onion, finely chopped

1 cup broccoli florets

1 cup sliced shiitake mushrooms

1 garlic clove, minced

8 large eggs, beaten

½ teaspoon sea salt

½ cup grated Parmesan cheese

PER SERVING Calories: 280; Total Fat: 21g; Saturated Fat: 6g; Sodium: 654mg; Carbohydrates: 7g; Fiber: 2g; Protein: 19g

1. Preheat the oven broiler on high.

2. In a medium ovenproof skillet over medium-high heat, heat the olive oil until it shimmers.

3. Add the onion, broccoli, and mushrooms, and cook, stirring occasionally, until the vegetables start to brown, about 5 minutes. Add the garlic and cook, stirring constantly, for 30 seconds. Arrange the vegetables in an even layer on the bottom of the pan.

4. While the vegetables cook, in a small bowl, whisk together the eggs and salt. Carefully pour the eggs over the vegetables. Cook without stirring, allowing the eggs to set around the vegetables. As the eggs begin to set around the edges, use a spatula to pull the edges away from the sides of the pan. Tilt the pan and allow the uncooked eggs to run into the spaces. Cook 1 to 2 minutes more, until it sets around the edges. The eggs will still be runny on top.

5. Sprinkle with the Parmesan and place the pan in the broiler. Broil until brown and puffy, about 3 minutes.

6. Cut into wedges to serve.

STORAGE NOTE: Frittatas reheat nicely, and they taste good cold, as well. Store frittata wedges in a resealable bag in the refrigerator for up to 3 days.

RECIPE TIP: This is a low-carb, high-fiber, high-protein breakfast. If you need some extra carbs, you may want to add yogurt or milk, a bread product, or fresh fruit. Be sure to consider the extra carb grams and adjust your insulin.

CANADIAN BACON AND EGG MUFFIN CUPS

≤10 · GLUTEN-FREE · NUT-FREE

SERVES 6 · PREP TIME: 5 MINUTES · COOK TIME: 20 MINUTES

Serve the whole family breakfast with this simple recipe that also does well on the go. It takes about 20 minutes to cook, but most of the time is waiting for the eggs to set in the oven. The Dijon mustard and hot sauce make these high-protein "muffins" super flavorful. You can vary the recipe by adding any chopped, sautéed veggies you like for even more flavor. Try red bell pepper or zucchini.

Cooking spray (for greasing)

6 large slices Canadian bacon

12 large eggs, beaten

1 teaspoon Dijon mustard

½ teaspoon sea salt

Dash hot sauce

1 cup shredded Swiss cheese

PER SERVING Calories: 259; Total Fat: 17g; Saturated Fat: 7g; Sodium: 781mg; Carbohydrates: 3g; Fiber: 0g; Protein: 24g

1. Preheat the oven to 350°F. Spray 6 nonstick muffin cups with cooking spray.

2. Line each cup with 1 slice of Canadian bacon.

3. In a bowl, whisk together the eggs, mustard, salt, and hot sauce. Fold in the cheese. Spoon the mixture into the muffin cups.

4. Bake until the eggs set, about 20 minutes.

STORAGE NOTE: Store extras in a resealable bag in the refrigerator for up to 3 days. Reheat in the microwave.

RECIPE TIP: This breakfast is very low-carb. If you need a few carbs, serve it with some plain Greek yogurt and sliced strawberries. Check the carb counts on your yogurt and remember to also consider the carbohydrate counts if you add berries or any fresh fruit (¾ cup of berries is approximately 15 grams carbohydrates).

SAUSAGE AND PEPPER BREAKFAST BURRITO

≤15 · NUT-FREE · ONE-POT

SERVES 4 · PREP TIME: 10 MINUTES · COOK TIME: 15 MINUTES

Sometimes you just want a burrito, even for breakfast. These breakfast burritos come together quickly, and you can easily customize their flavors by replacing breakfast sausage with an equal amount of chorizo, adding jalapeños, or changing the type of cheese you use. They make a great weekend family breakfast.

8 ounces bulk pork breakfast sausage

½ onion, chopped

1 green bell pepper, seeded and chopped

8 large eggs, beaten

4 (6-inch) low-carb tortillas

1 cup shredded pepper Jack cheese

½ cup sour cream (optional, for serving)

½ cup prepared salsa (optional, for serving)

STORAGE NOTE: Store the eggs separate from the cheese and tortillas in a tightly sealed container in the refrigerator for up to 3 days. Reheat in the microwave and assemble before serving.

PER SERVING Calories: 486; Total Fat: 36g; Saturated Fat: 14g; Sodium: 810mg; Carbohydrates: 13g; Fiber: 8g; Protein: 32g

1. In a large nonstick skillet on medium-high heat, cook the sausage, crumbling it with a spoon, until browned, about 5 minutes. Add the onion and bell pepper. Cook, stirring, until the veggies are soft, about 3 minutes. Add the eggs and cook, stirring, until eggs are set, about 3 minutes more.

2. Spoon the egg mixture onto the 4 tortillas. Top each with the cheese and fold into a burrito shape.

3. Serve with sour cream and salsa, if desired.

RECIPE TIP: If you're looking to add more carbohydrates, use regular tortillas instead of low-carb tortillas. Also, for added flavor, mash 1 avocado with the juice of 1 lime, ½ teaspoon salt, 1 minced garlic clove, ¼ cup finely diced red onion, and 2 tablespoons of chopped fresh cilantro. This makes four servings of guacamole and adds a bit more calories, fiber, and carbohydrates.

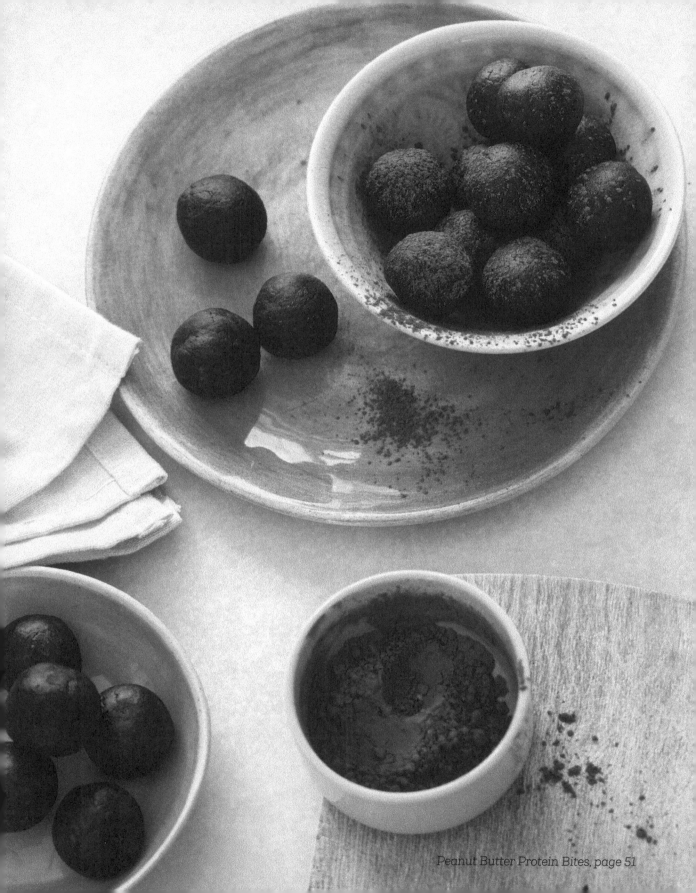

Peanut Butter Protein Bites, page 51

CHAPTER FOUR

Snacks

GARLIC KALE CHIPS

DAIRY-FREE · GLUTEN-FREE · NUT-FREE · VEGAN

SERVES 1 · PREP TIME: 5 MINUTES · COOK TIME: 15 MINUTES

If you're looking for a healthy alternative to chips, try these tasty low-carb, lightly crisp chips. Kale chips also contain calcium and are easy to tote along in a resealable container. Check out your local grocer or farmers' market to find fresh kale, and give these fun snacking chips a try.

1 (8-ounce) bunch kale, trimmed and cut into 2-inch pieces
1 tablespoon extra-virgin olive oil
½ teaspoon sea salt
¼ teaspoon garlic powder
Pinch cayenne (optional, to taste)

PER SERVING Calories: 231; Total Fat: 15g; Saturated Fat: 2g; Sodium: 678mg; Carbohydrates: 20g; Fiber: 4g; Protein: 7g

1. Preheat the oven to 350°F. Line two baking sheets with parchment paper.

2. Wash the kale and pat it completely dry.

3. In a large bowl, toss the kale with the olive oil, sea salt, garlic powder, and cayenne, if using.

4. Spread the kale in a single layer on the prepared baking sheets.

5. Bake until crisp, 12 to 15 minutes, rotating the sheets once.

STORAGE NOTE: Store baked kale chips in a plastic or glass container at room temperature for up to 5 days.

RECIPE TIP: It's easy to change flavors here; add ½ teaspoon of sesame oil, ¼ teaspoon of ground ginger, and 2 tablespoons of sesame seeds to the recipe and toss with the kale for an Asian flavor profile. This adds 2 grams of carbs and 1 gram of fiber.

PEANUT BUTTER PROTEIN BITES

≤10 · DAIRY-FREE · GLUTEN-FREE · VEGAN

MAKES 16 BALLS · PREP TIME: 10 MINUTES · COOK TIME: NONE

Easy to carry to the office or to school, these peanut butter bites provide a great low-carbohydrate snack with only 2 grams of carbohydrates. Double your peanut butter pleasure with sugar-free peanut butter protein powder (you can find it with other protein powders at the grocery store) and sugar-free peanut butter. If you can't find peanut butter protein powder, feel free to substitute any sugar-free, low-carb protein powder in vanilla, chocolate, or peanut butter, such as Vega protein powder.

½ cup sugar-free peanut butter

¾ cup (1 scoop) sugar-free peanut butter powder or sugar-free protein powder

2 tablespoons unsweetened cocoa powder

2 tablespoons canned coconut milk (or more to adjust consistency)

PER SERVING (1 ball) Calories: 61; Total Fat: 5g; Saturated Fat: 1g; Sodium: 19mg; Carbohydrates: 2g; Fiber: <1g; Protein: 4g

1. In a bowl, mix all ingredients until well combined.

2. Roll into 16 balls. Refrigerate before serving.

STORAGE NOTE: Store these in a resealable bag in the refrigerator for up to 5 days or in the freezer for up to 6 months.

RECIPE TIP: The great thing about these is that they're small. Adding 2 tablespoons of dried fruit, such as raisins or dried blueberries, will add carbohydrates. This may be an especially good choice before or after exercise, but if adding, be sure to consider the carbohydrate count in the dried fruits.

CINNAMON TOASTED PUMPKIN SEEDS

≤10 · DAIRY-FREE · GLUTEN-FREE · NUT-FREE · VEGAN

SERVES 4 · PREP TIME: 5 MINUTES · COOK TIME: 45 MINUTES

These flavorful pumpkin seeds require 45 minutes in the oven, but planning the night before will provide you with a healthy snack to enjoy on the run. Most pumpkin seeds come in savory or spicy mixes, but they have an earthy flavor that lends itself well to sweet spices, like cinnamon, as well. Pumpkin seeds are a great source of healthy fats, fiber, calcium, and potassium, and they are relatively low in carbs, which makes them a great snack.

1 cup pumpkin seeds

2 tablespoons canola oil

1 teaspoon cinnamon

2 (1-gram) packets stevia

¼ teaspoon sea salt

PER SERVING Calories: 135; Total Fat: 10g; Saturated Fat: 1g; Sodium: 76mg; Carbohydrates: 9g; Fiber: 1g; Protein: 3g

1. Preheat the oven to 300°F.

2. In a bowl, toss the pumpkin seeds with the oil, cinnamon, stevia, and salt.

3. Spread the seeds in a single layer on a rimmed baking sheet. Bake until browned and fragrant, stirring once or twice, about 45 minutes.

STORAGE NOTE: Store these in a resealable bag at room temperature for up to a week.

RECIPE TIP: You can also make a savory version, by replacing the cinnamon and stevia with 1 teaspoon of garlic powder and increasing the salt to ½ teaspoon. Serve these seeds sprinkled over half an avocado, if desired.

COCOA COATED ALMONDS

≤10 · DAIRY-FREE · GLUTEN-FREE · VEGAN

SERVES 4 · PREP TIME: 5 MINUTES · COOK TIME: 15 MINUTES

If you're looking for a sweet chocolate delight, look no further than almonds and cocoa powder. This delicious, healthy snack is filled with calcium and protein, keeps well, and has a satisfying crunch. If you're a chocolate fan, this is sure to become a favorite snack!

1 cup almonds

1 tablespoon cocoa powder

2 packets powdered stevia

PER SERVING Calories: 209; Total Fat: 18g; Saturated Fat: 1g; Sodium: 1mg; Carbohydrates: 9g; Fiber: 5g; Protein: 8g

1. Preheat the oven to 350°F. Line a baking sheet with parchment paper.

2. Spread the almonds in a single layer on the baking sheet. Bake for 5 minutes.

3. While the almonds bake, in a small bowl, mix the cocoa and stevia well. Add the hot almonds to the bowl. Toss to combine.

4. Return the almonds to the baking sheet and bake until fragrant, about 5 minutes more.

STORAGE NOTE: These store well in a resealable bag at room temperature for up to a week.

RECIPE TIP: After removing the almonds from the oven for the first time, toss them with a tablespoon of honey before adding them to the cocoa powder, omitting the stevia. This adds 4 grams per serving of carbs to the almonds. To keep them vegan, replace the honey with agave nectar or pure maple syrup.

GUACAMOLE WITH JICAMA

≤10 · DAIRY-FREE · GLUTEN-FREE · NUT-FREE · VEGAN

SERVES 4 · PREP TIME: 5 MINUTES · COOK TIME: NONE

Finding an alternative for chips is not easy, but crunchy jicama stands in for them well. Jicama is high in fiber and has a slightly sweet flavor. It pairs extremely well with this simple guacamole. Enjoy this tasty guacamole as a snack or pair it with meat, tacos, or fish.

1 avocado, cut into cubes

Juice of ½ lime

2 tablespoons finely chopped red onion

2 tablespoons chopped fresh cilantro

1 garlic clove, minced

¼ teaspoon sea salt

1 cup sliced jicama

PER SERVING Calories: 73; Total Fat: 5g; Saturated Fat: 1g; Sodium: 77mg; Carbohydrates: 8g; Fiber: 5g; Protein: 1g

1. In a small bowl, combine the avocado, lime juice, onion, cilantro, garlic, and salt. Mash lightly with a fork.

2. Serve with the jicama for dipping.

STORAGE NOTE: You can store peeled avocado overnight in the refrigerator, but keep air from reaching it. Just place plastic wrap directly around the surface of the avocado in a bowl so no air touches it. Store for up to a day.

RECIPE TIP: Need a bit of extra energy? Replace the jicama with tortilla chips you make by cutting 4 corn tortillas into wedges, tossing them with 1 tablespoon of olive oil, and baking them in a 350°F oven until crisp, about 7 minutes. This adds 7 grams of carbs per serving. You can also add 1 small chopped tomato to the guacamole, which adds about a gram of carbs per serving.

CAPRESE SKEWERS

≤10 · GLUTEN-FREE · NUT-FREE · VEGETARIAN

SERVES 2 · PREP TIME: 5 MINUTES · COOK TIME: NONE

Make these skewers ahead and refrigerate them overnight. They travel well, so it's a great snack to take to work or school. These are especially delicious in the summer, when cherry tomatoes are in season and so much sweeter. You can also toss all the ingredients together in a bowl (rip the basil into smaller bites) and make a salad. With only 6 grams of carbohydrates, you may not need any insulin with this snack.

12 cherry tomatoes

12 basil leaves

8 (1-inch) pieces mozzarella cheese

¼ cup Italian Vinaigrette (page 135) (optional, for serving)

PER SERVING Calories: 338; Total Fat: 24g; Saturated Fat: 14g; Sodium: 672mg; Carbohydrates: 6g; Fiber: 1g; Protein: 25g

1. On each of 4 wooden skewers, thread the following: 1 tomato, 1 basil leaf, 1 piece of cheese, 1 tomato, 1 basil leaf, 1 piece of cheese, 1 basil leaf, 1 tomato.

2. Serve with the vinaigrette, if desired, for dipping.

STORAGE NOTE: Refrigerate the skewers in a sealed container for up to 3 days.

RECIPE TIP: Add pitted black olives to each skewer (two per skewer) for variety and flavor.

ZUCCHINI HUMMUS DIP WITH RED BELL PEPPERS

≤10 · DAIRY-FREE · GLUTEN-FREE · NUT-FREE · ONE-POT · VEGAN

SERVES 4 · PREP TIME: 10 MINUTES · COOK TIME: NONE

Traditional hummus is prepared with chickpeas. This creative recipe replaces the chickpeas with zucchini, which makes it much lower in calories and carbohydrates. Mix up a batch of this garlicky, delicious hummus in your blender or food processor, and serve it with slices of red bell pepper (or your other favorite non-starchy veggie) for dipping.

2 zucchini, chopped

3 garlic cloves

2 tablespoons extra-virgin olive oil

2 tablespoons tahini

Juice of 1 lemon

½ teaspoon sea salt

1 red bell pepper, seeded and cut into sticks

PER SERVING Calories: 121; Total Fat: 11g; Saturated Fat: 2g; Sodium: 156mg; Carbohydrates: 7g; Fiber: 3g; Protein: 2g

1. In a blender or food processor, combine the zucchini, garlic, olive oil, tahini, lemon juice, and salt. Blend until smooth.

2. Serve with the red bell pepper for dipping.

STORAGE NOTE: Store in a container in the refrigerator for up to 3 days.

RECIPE TIP: Any vegetables will be healthy for this dip, but keep in mind that certain vegetables, such as carrots and sugar snap peas, are a bit higher in carbohydrates. Choose low-carb vegetables, such as celery, cucumbers, or mushrooms. If you're missing the chickpea flavor or need higher carbs, you can replace 1 zucchini with ¼ cup of cooked, drained chickpeas. Or just add whole chickpeas to the snack (½ cup chickpeas contains 15 grams of carbohydrates).

TURKEY ROLLUPS WITH VEGGIE CREAM CHEESE

≤10 · GLUTEN-FREE · NUT-FREE · ONE-POT

SERVES 2 · PREP TIME: 10 MINUTES · COOK TIME: NONE

These travel well, and you can assemble them a few days in advance. If you double or triple the recipe, you can take some with you to work or send them in lunch bags. The veggie cream cheese has nice flavor and a satisfying crunch. For even more crunch, wrap each piece of turkey in a large lettuce or kale leaf.

¼ cup cream cheese, at room temperature

2 tablespoons finely chopped red onion

2 tablespoons finely chopped red bell pepper

1 tablespoon chopped fresh chives

1 teaspoon Dijon mustard

1 garlic clove, minced

¼ teaspoon sea salt

6 slices deli turkey

PER SERVING Calories: 146; Total Fat: 10g; Saturated Fat: 6g; Sodium: 914mg; Carbohydrates: 5g; Fiber: 1g; Protein: 8g

1. In a small bowl, mix the cream cheese, red onion, bell pepper, chives, mustard, garlic, and salt.

2. Spread the mixture on the turkey slices and roll up.

STORAGE NOTE: Store in a container in the refrigerator for up to 3 days.

RECIPE TIP: Need a few more grams of carbs or a bit of crunch? Grate a carrot and roll it up with the turkey. One cup of raw vegetables has an estimated 5 grams of carbohydrates.

BUFFALO CHICKEN CELERY STICKS

≤10 · NUT-FREE · ONE-POT

SERVES 4 · PREP TIME: 10 MINUTES · COOK TIME: NONE

Like chicken wings? This portable version is easy to create, and it contains all the essential ingredients you get with Buffalo wings: blue cheese, hot sauce, chicken, and celery. Make these ahead, they'll keep, and they travel well. This is a great use of cooked chicken from the grocery store.

1 cup shredded cooked rotisserie
   chicken meat

¼ cup chunky blue cheese dressing

1 teaspoon Louisiana hot sauce

8 celery stalks, cut into halves lengthwise

PER SERVING Calories: 149; Total Fat: 12g; Saturated Fat: 2g; Sodium: 463mg; Carbohydrates: 3g; Fiber: 1g; Protein: 9g

1. In a small bowl, mix the chicken, blue cheese dressing, and hot sauce.

2. Spread the mixture into the celery stalks.

STORAGE NOTE: Store in a container in the refrigerator for up to 3 days.

RECIPE TIP: Children might love this as a celery stick, and adults may enjoy it as Buffalo chicken salad stuffed in an avocado.

VEGGIES WITH COTTAGE CHEESE RANCH DIP

≤10 · NUT-FREE · ONE-POT · VEGETARIAN

SERVES 4 · PREP TIME: 10 MINUTES · COOK TIME: NONE

Using cottage cheese as a base for ranch dip makes this snack higher in protein and heartier than if you made a mayo/buttermilk-based dip. Make the dip ahead of time and refrigerate it overnight if you want it super flavorful.

1 cup cottage cheese

2 tablespoons mayonnaise

Juice of ½ lemon

2 tablespoons chopped fresh chives

2 tablespoons chopped fresh dill

2 scallions, white and green parts, finely chopped

1 garlic clove, minced

½ teaspoon sea salt

2 zucchinis, cut into sticks

8 cherry tomatoes

1. In a small bowl, mix the cottage cheese, mayonnaise, lemon juice, chives, dill, scallions, garlic, and salt.

2. Serve with the zucchini sticks and cherry tomatoes for dipping.

STORAGE NOTE: Store in a container in the refrigerator for up to 3 days.

RECIPE TIP: Consider serving this healthy dip with some pita bread or pita chips for a healthy lunch option. You can add zucchini slices and cherry tomatoes to give it more volume, fiber, and crunch.

PER SERVING Calories: 90; Total Fat: 4g; Saturated Fat: 1g; Sodium: 387mg; Carbohydrates: 7g; Fiber: 1g; Protein: 7g

BAKED PARMESAN CRISPS

≤10 · GLUTEN-FREE · NUT-FREE · ONE-POT · VEGETARIAN

SERVES 2 · PREP TIME: 5 MINUTES · COOK TIME: 5 MINUTES

The sky's the limit—serve these crisps with the cottage cheese ranch dip (see page 59), with guacamole (see page 54), or just as they are. You can make as many as you like, and there's an easy microwave variation: Spread the cheese on parchment paper and microwave on high for about 2 minutes or until browned.

1 cup grated Parmesan cheese

STORAGE NOTE: These can be stored at room temperature for up to a week in a resealable bag.

PER SERVING Calories: 216; Total Fat: 14g; Saturated Fat: 9g; Sodium: 765mg; Carbohydrates: 2g; Fiber: 0g; Protein: 19g

1. Preheat the oven to 400°F. Line a rimmed baking sheet with parchment paper.

2. Spread the Parmesan on the prepared baking sheet into 4 mounds, spreading each mound out so it is flat but not touching the others.

3. Bake until brown and crisp, 3 to 5 minutes.

4. Cool for 5 minutes. Use a spatula to remove to a plate to continue cooling.

RECIPE TIP: These Parmesan chips may look like a high-carb chip, but since are made with only Parmesan cheese, they are quite the opposite. You may even need to add a breadstick or a dipping sauce if you're counting on the carbohydrates or using the dish to prevent low blood sugars. You could even spread them with the filling from the Buffalo Chicken Celery Sticks (page 58). They also make a great base for mini "pizzas" topped with some chopped pepperoni and a little tomato sauce.

ALMOND MILK NUT BUTTER MOCHA SMOOTHIE

≤15 · DAIRY-FREE · GLUTEN-FREE · ONE-POT · VEGAN

SERVES 1 · PREP TIME: 5 MINUTES · COOK TIME: NONE

This is a healthy alternative and has fewer carbohydrates than many of the smoothies you find in the marketplace. It also contains more calcium with much less simple sugar. If you love coffee drinks, this T1D-friendly version will surely please. This recipe calls for almond butter, but you can use any variety of nut butter, such as cashew, soy, or peanut butter. Check carbohydrate counts as you vary the recipe.

1 cup almond milk

2 tablespoons almond butter

1 tablespoon cocoa powder

1 teaspoon espresso powder (or to taste)

1 to 2 (1-gram) packets stevia (or to taste)

¼ teaspoon almond extract

½ cup crushed ice

PER SERVING Calories: 242; Total Fat: 21g; Saturated Fat: 2g; Sodium: 66mg; Carbohydrates: 12g; Fiber: 6g; Protein: 10g

In a blender, combine all of the ingredients and blend on high until smooth.

RECIPE TIP: For fewer carbs, you can reduce the nut butter to 1 tablespoon (almond butter has 3 grams of carbs per tablespoon). You can also add up to 1 cup of chopped kale with stems removed (7 grams carbs, 1 gram fiber) or baby spinach (1 gram carbs, 0.7 gram fiber) to add some greens and a few grams of carbs without affecting the taste or texture.

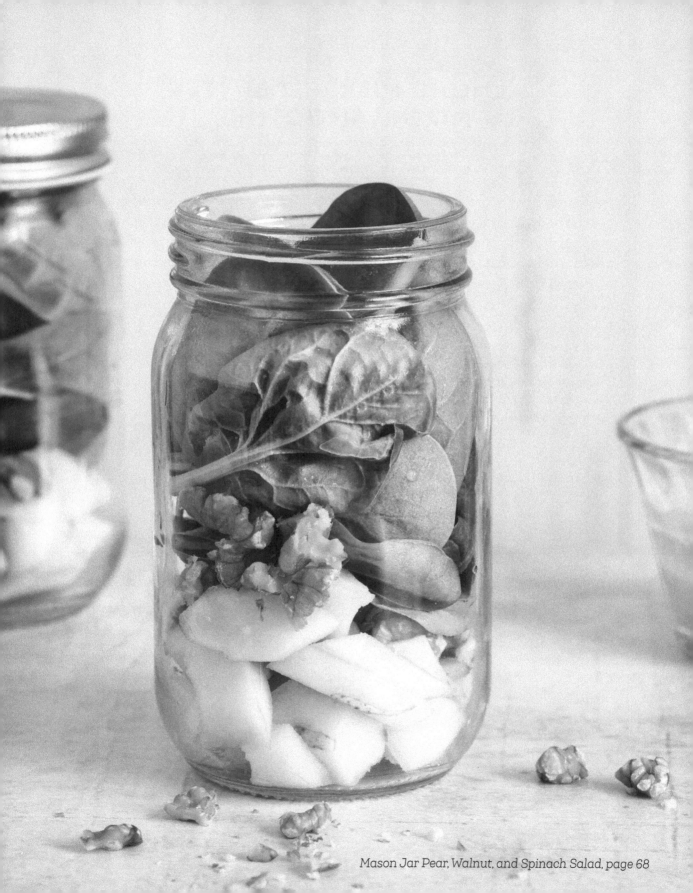

Mason Jar Pear, Walnut, and Spinach Salad, page 68

CHAPTER FIVE

Packable Lunches

LENTIL VEGETABLE SOUP

DAIRY-FREE · GLUTEN-FREE · NUT-FREE · ONE-POT · VEGAN

SERVES 4 · PREP TIME: 10 MINUTES · COOK TIME: 15 MINUTES

Lentil soup travels and reheats well. You can reheat it over medium-high heat on the stove top or in the microwave for a minute or two depending on the microwave's power. The soup is flavorful with fragrant rosemary and garlic. It's also a good source of iron and fiber, and beans have a low glycemic index. Choose an unsalted broth and add your own salt to adjust seasoning levels.

2 tablespoons extra-virgin olive oil

1 onion, finely chopped

1 carrot, chopped

1 cup chopped kale (stems removed)

3 garlic cloves, minced

1 cup canned lentils, drained and rinsed

5 cups unsalted vegetable broth

2 teaspoons dried rosemary (or 1 tablespoon chopped fresh rosemary)

½ teaspoon sea salt

¼ teaspoon freshly ground black pepper

PER SERVING Calories: 160; Total Fat: 7g; Saturated Fat: 1g; Sodium: 187mg; Carbohydrates: 19g; Fiber: 6g; Protein: 6g

1. In a large pot over medium-high heat, heat the olive oil until it shimmers. Add the onion and carrot and cook, stirring, until the vegetables begin to soften, about 3 minutes. Add the kale and cook for 3 minutes more. Add the garlic and cook, stirring constantly, for 30 seconds.

2. Stir in the lentils, vegetable broth, rosemary, salt, and pepper. Bring to a simmer. Simmer, stirring occasionally, for 5 minutes more.

STORAGE NOTE: This freezes well. Store it in 1½-cup servings in the freezer for up to 3 months or in the refrigerator for up to 5 days.

RECIPE TIP: Lentils are a low-glycemic carb that brings blood sugars up slowly. You can replace the lentils with 8 ounces of finely chopped mushrooms (cook them with the onion and carrot) to lower carb counts. If you need more carbs, you can add the entire can of lentils. When adjusting the recipe, remember to consider how much you are varying the carbohydrate count so you can bolus correctly.

EGG SALAD WRAPS

DAIRY-FREE · GLUTEN-FREE · NUT-FREE · ONE-POT · VEGETARIAN

SERVES 2 · PREP TIME: 10 MINUTES · COOK TIME: NONE

Many grocery stores sell hard-cooked eggs now, but it's easy to make your own. Place them in the bottom of a pan and cover them with about an inch of water. Put the pot on the stove on high and bring it to a boil. Turn off the heat, cover, and allow the eggs to sit for 14 minutes. Shock in ice water to stop the cooking, and then peel.

3 tablespoons mayonnaise

1 teaspoon Dijon mustard

1 tablespoon chopped fresh dill

½ teaspoon sea salt

¼ teaspoon paprika

4 hard-boiled large eggs, chopped

1 cup shelled fresh peas

2 tablespoons finely chopped red onion

2 large kale leaves

PER SERVING Calories: 295; Total Fat: 18g; Saturated Fat: 4g; Sodium: 620mg; Carbohydrates: 18g; Fiber: 4g; Protein: 17g

1. In a medium bowl, whisk together the mayonnaise, mustard, dill, salt, and paprika.

2. Stir in the eggs, peas, and onion.

3. Serve wrapped in kale leaves.

STORAGE NOTE: Egg salad will keep in the refrigerator for up to 3 days. Store the kale leaves and egg salad separately and wrap just before you eat them.

RECIPE TIP: For a lower-carbohydrate version, omit the peas and add 1 finely chopped celery stalk, which may reduce carbohydrates by as much as 15 grams. If you need to add carbohydrates, wrap the egg salad in a tortilla or whole-grain pita, or add a high-fiber cracker.

PIZZA STUFFED PITA

NUT-FREE · ONE-POT

SERVES 2 · PREP TIME: 10 MINUTES · COOK TIME: NONE

If you have an oven or microwave where you're headed, you can heat this up to melt the cheese (wrapped in foil in the oven at 350° for 10 minutes), but you can also enjoy it cold. It gives you all the flavors of pizza in a convenient pita pocket. Feel free to replace pepperoni with Canadian bacon or add red bell peppers or other chopped non-starchy veggies to change the flavor profile.

½ cup tomato sauce

½ teaspoon oregano

½ teaspoon garlic powder

½ cup chopped black olives

2 canned artichoke hearts, drained and chopped

2 ounces pepperoni, chopped

½ cup shredded mozzarella cheese

1 whole-wheat pita, halved

1. In a medium bowl, stir together the tomato sauce, oregano, and garlic powder.

2. Add the olives, artichoke hearts, pepperoni, and cheese. Stir to mix.

3. Spoon the mixture into the pita halves.

STORAGE NOTE: Store the filling and pita halves separately and spoon the mixture in just before serving. The filling will keep in the refrigerator for up to 3 days.

RECIPE TIP: For a fresh taste, add 10 halved cherry tomatoes to the mixture. For fewer carbs, scoop the mixture into a large spinach or lettuce leaf instead of the pita, or you can use a 6-inch low-carb tortilla for each serving.

PER SERVING Calories: 376; Total Fat: 23g; Saturated Fat: 8g; Sodium: 1076mg; Carbohydrates: 27g; Fiber: 6g; Protein: 17g

ALMOND BUTTER APPLE PITA POCKETS

DAIRY-FREE · ONE-POT · VEGAN

SERVES 2 · PREP TIME: 10 MINUTES · COOK TIME: NONE

Pita pockets are great for packable lunches because you can stuff all sorts of fillings in a pita, which serves as a handy container. These pitas are an updated and slightly more grown-up (lower-sugar) take on the classic PB&J, but the apples add a satisfying crunch and make this lunch high in soluble fiber.

½ apple, cored and chopped

¼ cup almond butter

½ teaspoon cinnamon

1 whole-wheat pita, halved

PER SERVING Calories: 313; Total Fat: 20g; Saturated Fat: 2g; Sodium: 174mg; Carbohydrates: 31g; Fiber: 7g; Protein: 8g

1. In a medium bowl, stir together the apple, almond butter, and cinnamon.

2. Spread with a spoon into the pita pocket halves.

STORAGE NOTE: You can store these in the refrigerator for up to 3 days, but they're best if they're made the day you're planning to eat them.

RECIPE TIP: For additional carbs and some texture, add some raw vegetables or a fresh fruit, but remember to calculate the carbohydrate grams in the total meal. Most fruits have 15 grams of carbs per serving, while 1 cup of raw vegetables will add 5 grams of carbs.

MASON JAR PEAR, WALNUT, AND SPINACH SALAD

≤10 · DAIRY-FREE · GLUTEN-FREE · VEGAN

SERVES 2 · PREP TIME: 10 MINUTES · COOK TIME: NONE

Preplanning for a healthy salad for lunch or dinner? Using a mason jar provides a pretty presentation and an excellent way for you to enjoy vegetables. It's a super quick way to put together a really flavorful salad. Store the dressing separately, and add it just before serving so you don't make your spinach soggy.

4 cups baby spinach

½ pear, cored, peeled, and chopped

¼ cup whole walnuts, chopped

2 tablespoons apple cider vinegar

2 tablespoons extra-virgin olive oil

1 teaspoon peeled and grated fresh ginger

½ teaspoon Dijon mustard

½ teaspoon sea salt

PER SERVING Calories: 254; Total Fat: 23g; Saturated Fat: 3g; Sodium: 340mg; Carbohydrates: 10g; Fiber: 4g; Protein: 4g

1. Layer the spinach on the bottom of two mason jars. Top with the pear and walnuts.

2. In a small bowl, whisk together the vinegar, oil, ginger, mustard, and salt. Put in another lidded container.

3. Shake the dressing before serving and add it to the mason jars. Close the jars and shake to distribute the dressing.

STORAGE NOTE: This salad will store for up to 3 days in the refrigerator. The vinaigrette will store in the refrigerator for up to a week.

RECIPE TIP: Need a few more grams of carbs for energy? Add a piece of whole-grain bread and remember to weigh the bread or look at the nutrition facts label to understand total carb content.

GREEK SALAD WITH FETA AND OLIVES

≤15 · GLUTEN-FREE · NUT-FREE · ONE-POT · VEGETARIAN

SERVES 4 · PREP TIME: 15 MINUTES · COOK TIME: NONE

Greek salad is like a flavor explosion. From the buttery olives to the grassy bite of feta to the fragrant herbs in the vinaigrette, it's a tasty salad that tends to be low in carbohydrates. Add whole-grain breadsticks, pita, or stuffed grape leaves if you want to add more carbs. Count the added rice in the grape leaves. To keep salad crisp, mix in the dressing just before serving.

4 cups chopped iceberg lettuce

1 cucumber, chopped

10 cherry tomatoes, halved

1 cup crumbled feta cheese

1 cup pitted black olives

½ red onion, thinly sliced

½ cup Greek Vinaigrette (page 135)

PER SERVING Calories: 337; Total Fat: 29g; Saturated Fat: 9g; Sodium: 904mg; Carbohydrates: 13g; Fiber: 3g; Protein: 8g

1. In a large bowl, combine the lettuce, cucumber, tomatoes, feta, olives, and onion. Toss to combine.

2. Toss with the dressing just before serving.

STORAGE NOTE: This salad will store for up to 3 days in the refrigerator. The vinaigrette will store in the refrigerator for up to a week.

RECIPE TIP: Add some whole-wheat croutons for crunch and to boost carbs; ¼ cup of whole-wheat croutons adds 15 grams of carbs.

ASIAN CHICKEN SLAW

DAIRY-FREE · GLUTEN-FREE · NUT-FREE · ONE-POT

SERVES 2 · PREP TIME: 10 MINUTES · COOK TIME: NONE

Slaw is not just an appetizer; this dish provides a healthy balance of carbs, proteins, and fats. This meal can be prepared with any leftover chicken, or you can buy a grocery store rotisserie chicken and shred the meat. Chicken freezes well and can be stored for 6 months. Thaw to make a quick, easy meal or appetizer.

1 cup shredded cooked rotisserie chicken meat

3 cups shredded cabbage or coleslaw mix

1 Asian pear, cored, peeled, and julienned

2 scallions, white and green parts, sliced on the bias (cut diagonally into thin slices)

¼ cup Asian Vinaigrette (page 134)

PER SERVING Calories: 297; Total Fat: 20g; Saturated Fat: 9g; Sodium: 392mg; Carbohydrates: 16g; Fiber: 5g; Protein: 16g

1. In a large bowl, combine the chicken, cabbage, pear, and scallions.

2. Toss with the vinaigrette just before serving.

STORAGE NOTE: The slaw will store for up to 3 days in the refrigerator. The vinaigrette will store in the refrigerator for up to a week.

RECIPE TIP: For fewer carbs, omit the pear and add an additional 1 cup of coleslaw mix or shredded cabbage. That will reduce carb counts by 14 grams per serving. To boost carbs, add ½ cup of chopped peanuts with the vinaigrette–this will increase carbs by 6 grams per serving.

EASY CHOP CHOP SALAD

DAIRY-FREE · GLUTEN-FREE · NUT-FREE · ONE-POT

SERVES 2 · PREP TIME: 10 MINUTES · COOK TIME: NONE

Chopped salads are fantastic because they are so easy to customize to your taste. Just chop up a bunch of different veggies, add some chopped meat, and toss with dressing, and you've got a tasty meal on the go. This version uses ham, but you can also use chicken or turkey if you wish, as well as any combo of non-starchy veggies.

2 cups chopped iceberg lettuce

10 cherry tomatoes, halved

1 cup pitted black olives, chopped

6 ounces ham, chopped

½ red onion, chopped

1 red bell pepper, seeded and chopped

10 basil leaves, torn

¼ cup Italian Vinaigrette (page 135)

PER SERVING Calories: 434; Total Fat: 31g; Saturated Fat: 7g; Sodium: 2285mg; Carbohydrates: 17g; Fiber: 5g; Protein: 22g

1. In a large bowl, combine the lettuce, tomatoes, olives, ham, onion, bell pepper, and basil leaves.

2. Toss with the vinaigrette just before serving.

STORAGE NOTE: The salad will store for up to 3 days in the refrigerator. The vinaigrette will store in the refrigerator for up to a week.

RECIPE TIP: Make this salad heartier by adding 4 ounces of chopped mozzarella cheese. You can also balance this chopped salad by adding a vegetarian source of protein and ½ cup of kidney beans, which would add 15 grams of carbs.

CHICKEN ZOODLE SOUP

≤15 · DAIRY-FREE · GLUTEN-FREE · NUT-FREE

SERVES 4 · PREP TIME: 10 MINUTES · COOK TIME: 15 MINUTES

Finding an alternative to noodles is easy—try zucchini noodles! The zoodle alternative is lower in carbohydrates, has fiber, and offers a slower blood sugar response than regular pasta.

2 tablespoons extra-virgin olive oil

12 ounces chicken breast, chopped

1 onion, chopped

2 carrots, chopped

2 celery stalks, chopped

2 garlic cloves

6 cups unsalted chicken broth

1 teaspoon dried thyme

1 teaspoon sea salt

2 medium zucchinis, cut into noodles (or store-bought zucchini noodles)

STORAGE NOTE: This freezes well. Store it for up to 6 months in 1½-cup servings in the freezer. Store it for up to 3 days in the refrigerator.

PER SERVING Calories: 236; Total Fat: 10g; Saturated Fat: 2g; Sodium: 201mg; Carbohydrates: 11g; Fiber: 3g; Protein: 27g

1. In a large pot over medium-high heat, heat the olive oil until it shimmers. Add the chicken and cook until it is opaque, about 5 minutes. With a slotted spoon, remove the chicken from the pot and set aside on a plate.

2. Add the onion, carrots, and celery to the pot. Cook, stirring occasionally, until the vegetables are soft, about 5 minutes. Add the garlic and cook, stirring constantly, for 30 seconds. Add the chicken broth, thyme, and salt. Bring to a boil, and reduce the heat to medium.

3. Add the zucchini and return the chicken to the pan, adding any juices that have collected on the plate. Cook, stirring occasionally, until the zucchini noodles are soft, 1 to 2 minutes more.

RECIPE TIP: Using zucchini in place of noodles makes this a very-low-carb soup. For a heartier, higher-carb soup, you can add 2 ounces of dried buckwheat noodles, which will add 43 grams of carbs and 3 grams of fiber per serving. The noodles will need to simmer for 5 to 8 minutes—check the package for nutrition information and cooking instructions.

CURRIED TUNA SALAD LETTUCE WRAPS

DAIRY-FREE · NUT-FREE · ONE-POT

SERVES 2 · PREP TIME: 10 MINUTES · COOK TIME: NONE

Water chestnuts add a delicious crunch to tuna salad and a mild nutty flavor to these Asian-themed tuna wraps. You can find canned water chestnuts in the Asian section of your local grocery store. Just drain and chop them before adding them to your tuna salad. This is a uniquely crunchy wrap you're sure to love.

⅓ cup mayonnaise

1 tablespoon freshly squeezed lemon juice

1 teaspoon curry powder

1 teaspoon reduced-sodium soy sauce

½ teaspoon sriracha (or to taste)

½ cup canned water chestnuts, drained and chopped

2 (2.6-ounce) package tuna packed in water, drained

2 large butter lettuce leaves

PER SERVING Calories: 271; Total Fat: 14g; Saturated Fat: 2g; Sodium: 627mg; Carbohydrates: 18g; Fiber: 3g; Protein: 19g

1. In a medium bowl, whisk together the mayonnaise, lemon juice, curry powder, soy sauce, and sriracha.

2. Add the water chestnuts and tuna. Stir to combine.

3. Serve wrapped in the lettuce leaves.

STORAGE NOTE: Store the tuna salad for up to 3 days in the refrigerator.

RECIPE TIP: If you need a few more carbs, you can serve this with ½ slice of whole-wheat naan (Indian flatbread) per serving on the side. Be sure to look at the carbohydrate counts when adding any breads or crackers. This recipe also works nicely scooped into half an avocado.

ROAST BEEF AND SPINACH WRAPS WITH CHIMICHURRI CREAM CHEESE

NUT-FREE · ONE-POT

SERVES 2 · PREP TIME: 10 MINUTES · COOK TIME: NONE

Chimichurri sauce is like pesto, and mixing it with softened cream cheese seems the perfect way to add it to some tasty roast beef. Beef and Chimichurri make a classic flavor combination, elevated further with the bite of garlic, savory flavors of fresh herbs, and a bright acidity from the lemon.

¼ cup softened cream cheese
¼ cup Chimichurri (page 129)
2 (6-inch) low-carb tortillas
1 cup baby spinach
½ tomato, chopped
6 ounces thinly sliced roast beef

PER SERVING Calories: 361; Total Fat: 25g; Saturated Fat: 9g; Sodium: 255mg; Carbohydrates: 16g; Fiber: 8g; Protein: 29g

1. In a small bowl, mix the cream cheese and Chimichurri.

2. Spread the mixture on the tortillas.

3. Top each with the spinach, tomato, and roast beef. Roll and cut in half.

STORAGE NOTE: This will store wrapped in plastic or in a resealable bag for 2 days in the refrigerator.

RECIPE TIP: If you want to reduce carbohydrates, use large spinach or kale leaves instead of low-carb tortillas. If you want to add carbs, use regular tortilla wraps.

SPICY CORN AND SHRIMP SALAD IN AVOCADO

DAIRY-FREE · GLUTEN-FREE · NUT-FREE · ONE-POT

SERVES 2 · PREP TIME: 10 MINUTES · COOK TIME: NONE

An avocado half makes the perfect vehicle for a spicy shrimp, corn, and bell pepper salad. Its creamy texture goes well with the crisp corn and bell peppers, and it's a good source of healthy fats. Plus, the briny shrimp just tastes delicious when combined with earthy corn, sweet bell peppers, and grassy avocados.

¼ cup mayonnaise

1 teaspoon sriracha (or to taste)

½ teaspoon lemon zest

¼ teaspoon sea salt

4 ounces cooked baby shrimp

½ cup cooked and cooled corn kernels

½ red bell pepper, seeded and chopped

1 avocado, halved lengthwise

PER SERVING Calories: 326; Total Fat: 21g; Saturated Fat: 3g; Sodium: 538mg; Carbohydrates: 25g; Fiber: 7g; Protein: 15g

1. In a medium bowl, combine the mayonnaise, sriracha, lemon zest, and salt.

2. Add the shrimp, corn, and bell pepper. Mix to combine.

3. Spoon the mixture into the avocado halves.

STORAGE NOTE: The shrimp salad will keep for up to 3 days in the refrigerator. Don't cut the avocado until you're ready to serve.

RECIPE TIP: Corn is considered a starch, with similar amounts of carbohydrates as peas or pasta—½ cup corn has 15 grams of carbs. Depending on your carb needs, add or subtract corn in this easy recipe.

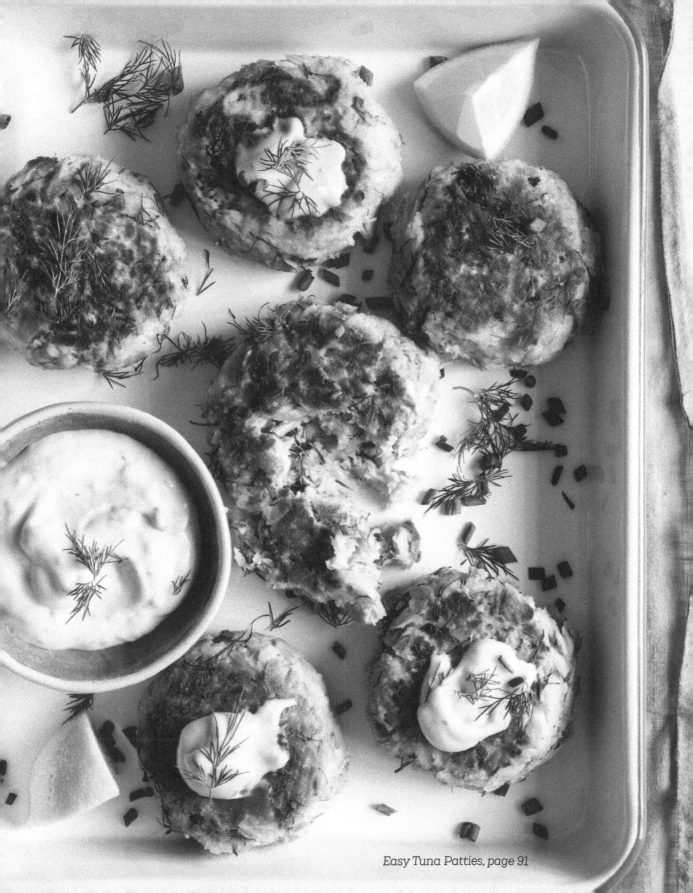

Easy Tuna Patties, page 91

CHAPTER SIX

Meatless and Seafood Mains

SPINACH MINI CRUSTLESS QUICHES

≤10 · GLUTEN-FREE · NUT-FREE · VEGETARIAN

SERVES 6 · PREP TIME: 10 MINUTES · COOK TIME: 15 MINUTES

Miniaturizing quiches in a muffin tin is a great way to speed up cooking time while still delivering all the savory flavors of a quiche. You can add more veggies to these quiches or serve them with a side salad for a healthy extra dose of vegetables. This dish is a good source of protein and iron.

Nonstick cooking spray

2 tablespoons extra-virgin olive oil

1 onion, finely chopped

2 cups baby spinach

2 garlic cloves, minced

8 large eggs, beaten

¼ cup whole milk

½ teaspoon sea salt

¼ teaspoon freshly ground black pepper

1 cup shredded Swiss cheese

STORAGE NOTE: Quiches freeze well. Pop them out of the muffin tin and freeze them in resealable bags for up to 6 months, or store in the refrigerator for up to 3 days.

PER SERVING Calories: 218; Total Fat: 17g; Saturated Fat: 6g; Sodium: 237mg; Carbohydrates: 4g; Fiber: <1g; Protein: 14g

1. Preheat the oven to 375°F. Spray a 6-cup muffin tin with nonstick cooking spray.

2. In a large skillet over medium-high heat, heat the olive oil until it shimmers. Add the onion and cook until soft, about 4 minutes. Add the spinach and cook, stirring, until the spinach softens, about 1 minute. Add the garlic. Cook, stirring constantly, for 30 seconds. Remove from heat and let cool.

3. In a medium bowl, beat together the eggs, milk, salt, and pepper.

4. Fold the cooled vegetables and the cheese into the egg mixture. Spoon the mixture into the prepared muffin tins. Bake until the eggs are set, about 15 minutes. Allow to rest for 5 minutes before serving.

RECIPE TIP: This is a relatively low-carb meal. To boost carbs, serve with fresh fruit or soup. Thicker soups tend to have more carbohydrates than simple broths. Added carbs need to be accounted for, so you can bolus correctly.

BAKED EGG SKILLET WITH AVOCADO

DAIRY-FREE · GLUTEN-FREE · NUT-FREE · ONE-POT · VEGETARIAN

SERVES 4 · PREP TIME: 5 MINUTES · COOK TIME: 25 MINUTES

With its lovely Southwestern flavor profile, these eggs are great for breakfast, lunch, or a family dinner. You can add additional non-starchy veggies, such as spinach, kale, or red bell peppers, for additional vitamins and minerals. You can also replace the avocado with homemade guacamole (see page 54).

2 tablespoons extra-virgin olive oil

1 red onion, chopped

1 green bell pepper, seeded and chopped

1 sweet potato, cut into ½-inch pieces

1 teaspoon chili powder

½ teaspoon sea salt

4 large eggs

½ cup shredded pepper Jack cheese

1 avocado, cut into cubes

STORAGE NOTE: This won't keep well. Make it fresh and enjoy it right away.

PER SERVING Calories: 284; Total Fat: 21g; Saturated Fat: 6g; Sodium: 264mg; Carbohydrates: 16g; Fiber: 5g; Protein: 12g

1. Preheat the oven to 350°F.

2. In a large, ovenproof skillet over medium-high heat, heat the olive oil until it shimmers. Add the onion, bell pepper, sweet potato, chili powder, and salt, and cook, stirring occasionally, until the vegetables start to brown, about 10 minutes.

3. Remove from heat. Arrange the vegetables in the pan to form 4 wells. Crack an egg into each well. Sprinkle the cheese on the vegetables, around the edges of the eggs.

4. Bake until the eggs set, about 10 minutes.

5. Top with avocado before serving.

RECIPE TIP: For fewer carbs, you can replace the sweet potato with 1 cup of raw chopped carrots, which has only about 5 grams of carbs per serving. For a few extra grams of carbs, you can top each serving with 2 tablespoons of prepared salsa. Check the serving size and carbohydrate counts on the salsa, and look for products with less than 5 grams of sugar. You can also add chopped tomatoes to serve.

MINESTRONE

DAIRY-FREE · NUT-FREE · ONE-POT · VEGAN

SERVES 4 · PREP TIME: 10 MINUTES · COOK TIME: 20 MINUTES

Minestrone is a hearty vegetable soup with lots of flavor. Feel free to expand your veggie repertoire beyond what's listed here; just make sure you include the carb counts of any additional vegetables for your insulin calculations.

2 tablespoons extra-virgin olive oil

1 onion, chopped

1 red bell pepper, seeded and chopped

2 garlic cloves, minced

2 cups green beans (fresh or frozen; halved if fresh)

6 cups low-sodium vegetable broth

1 (14-ounce) can crushed tomatoes

1 tablespoon Italian seasoning

½ cup dried whole-wheat elbow macaroni

½ teaspoon sea salt

Pinch red pepper flakes (or to taste)

PER SERVING Calories: 200; Total Fat: 7g; Saturated Fat: 1g; Sodium: 477mg; Carbohydrates: 29g; Fiber: 7g; Protein: 5g

1. In a large pot over medium-high heat, heat the olive oil until it shimmers. Add the onion and bell pepper and cook, stirring occasionally, until they soften, about 3 minutes. Add the garlic and cook, stirring constantly, for 30 seconds. Add the green beans, vegetable broth, tomatoes, and Italian seasoning and bring to a boil.

2. Add the elbow macaroni, salt, and red pepper flakes. Cook, stirring occasionally, until the macaroni is soft, about 8 minutes.

STORAGE NOTE: Minestrone freezes well, so you can make a double batch and freeze it in 1½-cup servings for up to 6 months. It will keep refrigerated for up to 5 days.

RECIPE TIP: For fewer carbs, replace the elbow macaroni with 2 cups of chopped non-starchy vegetables, such as zucchini. That will eliminate about 10 grams of carbs per serving. For a few more carbs, add up to ½ cup of canned kidney beans, which have more fiber and carbs and a low glycemic effect—½ cup kidney beans is estimated at 15 grams of carbohydrates per serving.

ZOODLES WITH PEA PESTO

≤15 · GLUTEN-FREE · VEGETARIAN

SERVES 4 · PREP TIME: 10 MINUTES · COOK TIME: 10 MINUTES

Peas are a starchy vegetable but can easily fit into a healthy plan. This recipe works best with fresh peas, which have enough texture to hold up in pesto. You can also use shelled edamame in place of the peas here for additional protein and a slightly less-sweet flavor profile.

3 zucchinis
2 tablespoons extra-virgin olive oil
Pinch sea salt
Pea Pesto (page 128)

PER SERVING Calories: 348; Total Fat: 30g; Saturated Fat: 5g; Sodium: 343mg; Carbohydrates: 13g; Fiber: 1g; Protein: 10g

1. Using a vegetable peeler, cut the zucchini lengthwise into long strips. Use a knife to cut the strips into the desired width. Alternatively, use a spiralizer to cut the zucchini into noodles.

2. In a large skillet over medium-high heat, heat the olive oil until it shimmers. Add the zucchini and cook until it starts to soften, about 3 minutes. Add the sea salt.

3. Toss the zucchini noodles with the pesto.

STORAGE NOTE: Both the zucchini noodles and the pesto are best served right away.

RECIPE TIP: Butternut squash also makes great zoodles, and it's slightly higher in carbs. You can replace the zucchini noodles with butternut noodles (1 cup per serving), which have 16 grams of carbs and 3 grams of fiber per cup.

BUTTERNUT NOODLES WITH MUSHROOM SAUCE

DAIRY-FREE · GLUTEN-FREE · NUT-FREE · ONE-POT · VEGAN

SERVES 4 · PREP TIME: 10 MINUTES · COOK TIME: 20 MINUTES

Here's an excellent alternative to a high-carb pasta meal. Mushrooms add a hearty, earthy flavor to this butternut pasta. One butternut squash makes about 3 cups of noodles, so you'll need about a squash and a half for this recipe. You can use a spiralizer, buy the noodles precut in the produce section of the grocery store, or use a vegetable peeler and knife to cut the noodles. One cup of cooked butternut squash is estimated at 16 grams of carbohydrates and is a good source of fiber.

¼ cup extra-virgin olive oil

1 pound cremini mushrooms, sliced

½ red onion, finely chopped

1 teaspoon dried thyme

½ teaspoon sea salt

3 garlic cloves, minced

½ cup dry white wine

Pinch red pepper flakes

4 cups butternut noodles

4 ounces grated Parmesan cheese (optional, for serving)

STORAGE NOTE: Veggie noodles don't keep well once they're cooked, so it's best to make them fresh. You can make the sauce ahead, store that in the refrigerator for up to 3 days, reheat, and add the noodles.

1. In a large skillet over medium-high heat, heat the olive oil until it shimmers. Add the mushrooms, onion, thyme, and salt. Cook, stirring occasionally, until the mushrooms start to brown, about 6 minutes. Add the garlic and cook, stirring constantly, for 30 seconds. Add the white wine and red pepper flakes. Stir to combine.

2. Add the noodles. Cook, stirring occasionally, until the noodles are tender, about 5 minutes.

3. If desired, serve topped with grated Parmesan.

RECIPE TIP: Replacing the butternut squash with zucchini noodles or shirataki noodles (usually found in the produce section of the grocery store) will lower the carbohydrate count in this recipe. That's just a different twist on an already very healthy recipe.

PER SERVING Calories: 244; Total Fat: 14g; Saturated Fat: 2g; Sodium: 159mg; Carbohydrates: 22g; Fiber: 4g; Protein: 4g

TOFU VEGGIE STIR-FRY

DAIRY-FREE · GLUTEN-FREE · NUT-FREE · ONE-POT · VEGAN

SERVES 4 · PREP TIME: 10 MINUTES · COOK TIME: 20 MINUTES

Who needs takeout? This heart-healthy, high-fiber stir-fry is fragrant with ginger and garlic. The brown rice used here is higher in fiber and less processed than white rice. The rice is more for flavor rather than the bulk of the meal. To save time, you can find quick-cooking instant brown rice in the rice section of the grocery store.

3 tablespoons extra-virgin olive oil

4 scallions, sliced

12 ounces firm tofu, cut into ½-inch pieces

4 cups broccoli, broken into florets

4 garlic cloves, minced

1 teaspoon peeled and grated fresh ginger

¼ cup vegetable broth

2 tablespoons soy sauce (use gluten-free soy sauce if necessary)

1 cup cooked brown rice

PER SERVING Calories: 236; Total Fat: 13g; Saturated Fat: 2g; Sodium: 361mg; Carbohydrates: 21g; Fiber: 4g; Protein: 11g

1. In a large skillet over medium-high heat, heat the olive oil until it shimmers. Add the scallions, tofu, and broccoli and cook, stirring, until the vegetables begin to soften, about 6 minutes. Add the garlic and ginger and cook, stirring constantly, for 30 seconds.

2. Add the broth, soy sauce, and rice. Cook, stirring, 1 to 2 minutes more to heat the rice through.

STORAGE NOTE: Refrigerate in a sealed container for up to 5 days, or freeze for up to 6 months.

RECIPE TIP: You can reduce carbohydrates by replacing the brown rice with an equal amount of cauliflower rice. This reduces the carb count by approximately 10 grams. To make it, simply grate cauliflower using a box grater. Increase cooking time by a minute or two to allow the cauliflower to soften.

VEGGIE CHILI

DAIRY-FREE · NUT-FREE · ONE-POT · VEGAN

SERVES 4 · PREP TIME: 10 MINUTES · COOK TIME: 15 MINUTES

This combination of beans and vegetarian proteins is hearty and nutritious. In addition to the protein, it's packed with low-glycemic carbohydrates and contains calcium and iron. You can find veggie crumbles in the freezer section of many grocery stores, with other meat substitutes. Double-check the label for the exact grams of carbs per serving and take this into account if you vary this recipe.

2 tablespoons extra-virgin olive oil

1 onion, finely chopped

1 green bell pepper, seeded and chopped

2 (14-ounce) cans crushed tomatoes

1 (14-ounce) can kidney beans, drained and rinsed

2 cups veggie crumbles (such as MorningStar Farms Grillers Crumbles)

1 tablespoon chili powder

1 teaspoon garlic powder

½ teaspoon sea salt

In a large skillet over medium-high heat, heat the olive oil until it shimmers. Add the onion and bell pepper and cook, stirring occasionally, for 5 minutes. Add the tomatoes, beans, veggie crumbles, chili powder, garlic powder, and salt. Bring to a simmer, stirring. Reduce heat and cook for 5 minutes more, stirring occasionally.

STORAGE NOTE: Refrigerate in a sealed container for up to 3 days, or freeze for up to 6 months.

RECIPE TIP: Reduce carbs by about 11 grams per serving by reducing kidney beans to ½ a can. Add 4 cups of vegetable broth to make a chili soup.

PER SERVING Calories: 283; Total Fat: 10g; Saturated Fat: 1g; Sodium: 1130mg; Carbohydrates: 39g; Fiber: 13g; Protein: 17g

CIOPPINO

≤15 · DAIRY-FREE · GLUTEN-FREE · NUT-FREE · ONE-POT

SERVES 4 · PREP TIME: 10 MINUTES · COOK TIME: 20 MINUTES

Cioppino is a rich, fragrant, flavorful seafood soup or stew with a tomato base. This version uses only two types of seafood (shrimp and fish) to keep it simple, but you can add any other seafood you'd like for a heartier soup.

2 tablespoons extra-virgin olive oil

1 onion, finely chopped

1 garlic clove, minced

½ cup dry white wine

1 (14-ounce) can tomato sauce

8 ounces cod, pin bones removed, cut into 1-inch pieces

8 ounces shrimp, peeled and deveined

1 tablespoon Italian seasoning

½ teaspoon sea salt

Pinch red pepper flakes

PER SERVING Calories: 243; Total Fat: 8g; Saturated Fat: 1g; Sodium: 271mg; Carbohydrates: 11g; Fiber: 2g; Protein: 23g

1. In a large skillet over medium-high heat, heat the olive oil until it shimmers. Add the onion and cook, stirring occasionally, for 3 minutes. Add the garlic and cook, stirring constantly, for 30 seconds. Add the wine and cook, stirring, for 1 minute.

2. Add the tomato sauce. Bring to a simmer. Stir in the cod, shrimp, Italian seasoning, salt, and pepper flakes. Simmer until the fish is just opaque, about 5 minutes.

STORAGE NOTE: Refrigerate in a sealed container for up to 3 days, or freeze for up to 6 months.

RECIPE TIP: Add up to 1 cup of cooked white beans, such as cannellini beans, when you add the seafood. On average, ½ cup cooked beans will add 15 to 20 grams of carbohydrates.

Meatless and Seafood Mains **85**

QUICK CLAM CHOWDER

NUT-FREE · ONE-POT

SERVES 4 · PREP TIME: 10 MINUTES · COOK TIME: 15 MINUTES

Canned clams give a nice seafood flavor to this quick chowder. You can also use fresh clam meat, but you'll need to chop up the clams before adding them to the soup. The fennel adds lots of flavor here, with a slight anise flavor that pairs beautifully with the seafood. To make this dairy-free, use an unsweetened almond milk in place of the milk.

2 tablespoons extra-virgin olive oil

3 slices pepper bacon, chopped

1 onion, chopped

1 red bell pepper, seeded and chopped

1 fennel bulb, chopped

3 tablespoons flour

5 cups low-sodium or unsalted chicken broth

6 ounces chopped canned clams, undrained

½ teaspoon sea salt

½ cup milk

STORAGE NOTE: This will keep frozen for up to 6 months, or refrigerated for up to 3 days.

PER SERVING Calories: 335; Total Fat: 20g; Saturated Fat: 5g; Sodium: 496mg; Carbohydrates: 21g; Fiber: 3g; Protein: 20g

1. In a large pot over medium-high heat, heat the olive oil until it shimmers. Add the bacon and cook, stirring, until browned, about 4 minutes. Remove the bacon from the fat with a slotted spoon, and set it aside on a plate.

2. Add the onion, bell pepper, and fennel to the fat in the pot. Cook, stirring occasionally, until the vegetables are soft, about 5 minutes. Add the flour and cook, stirring constantly, for 1 minute. Add the broth, clams, and salt. Bring to a simmer. Cook, stirring, until the soup thickens, about 5 minutes more.

3. Stir in the milk and return the bacon to the pot. Cook, stirring, 1 minute more.

RECIPE TIP: If you need a few more grams of carbs, add chopped carrots and onions, and crumble in some crackers. General guideline: 1 ounce of crackers equals 15 grams of carbohydrates. All crackers are different, so look at the nutrition facts label or weigh on a digital scale.

SHRIMP PERI-PERI

≤15 · DAIRY-FREE · GLUTEN-FREE · NUT-FREE

SERVES 4 · PREP TIME: 10 MINUTES · COOK TIME: 15 MINUTES

Peri-Peri Sauce (also called piri-piri) is a spicy South African sauce you can enjoy on just about any type of protein, from shrimp to beef. This shrimp cooks quickly under the broiler, and the sauce is fragrant and flavorful without overpowering the inherently sweet, briny flavor of the shrimp.

Peri-Peri Sauce (page 130)
1 pound large shrimp, shelled and deveined
2 tablespoons extra-virgin olive oil
Sea salt

PER SERVING Calories: 279; Total Fat: 16g; Saturated Fat: 2g; Sodium: 464mg; Carbohydrates: 10g; Fiber: 3g; Protein: 24g

1. Preheat the oven broiler on high.

2. In a small pot, bring the Peri-Peri Sauce to a simmer.

3. Meanwhile, place the cleaned shrimp on a rimmed baking sheet, deveined-side down. Brush with the olive oil and sprinkle with the salt.

4. Broil until opaque, about 5 minutes. Serve with the sauce on the side for dipping or spooned over the top of the shrimp.

STORAGE NOTE: Cook this on demand. Store cooked shrimp separately from sauce for up to 3 days in the refrigerator.

RECIPE TIP: Serve this dish with a ¼-cup serving of cooked quinoa on the side (9 grams of carbs, 1 gram of fiber) and some steamed non-starchy veggies, such as broccoli.

COD WITH MANGO SALSA

≤15 · DAIRY-FREE · GLUTEN-FREE · NUT-FREE

SERVES 4 · PREP TIME: 10 MINUTES · COOK TIME: 10 MINUTES

Cod is a mild-flavored, low-fat, white-fleshed fish; you can replace with whatever whitefish is available in your area. Be sure to carefully remove any pin bones using a pair of needle-nose tweezers to pull the bones away from the flesh. The salsa complements the sweet flesh of the cod perfectly. Serve with vegetables and whole grains to create a balanced meal with the right number of carbs.

1 pound cod, cut into 4 fillets, pin
    bones removed

2 tablespoons extra-virgin olive oil

¾ teaspoon sea salt, divided

1 mango, pitted, peeled, and cut into cubes

¼ cup chopped cilantro

½ red onion, finely chopped

1 jalapeño, seeded and finely chopped

1 garlic clove, minced

Juice of 1 lime

PER SERVING Calories: 197; Total Fat: 8g; Saturated Fat: 1g; Sodium: 354mg; Carbohydrates: 13g; Fiber: 2g; Protein: 21g

1. Preheat the oven broiler on high.

2. On a rimmed baking sheet, brush the cod with the olive oil and season with ½ teaspoon of the salt. Broil until the fish is opaque, 5 to 10 minutes.

3. Meanwhile, in a small bowl, combine the mango, cilantro, onion, jalapeño, garlic, lime juice, and remaining ¼ teaspoon of salt.

4. Serve the cod with the salsa spooned over the top.

STORAGE NOTE: Cook this on demand. Store the cooked cod separately from the salsa for up to 3 days in the refrigerator.

RECIPE TIP: Reduce carbs by replacing the mango with 1 large chopped tomato. Serve this dish with a side salad and vinaigrette or a steamed non-starchy veggie. For more carbs, add steamed brown rice.

SCALLOP PO' BOY LETTUCE CUPS

DAIRY-FREE · NUT-FREE

SERVES 4 · PREP TIME: 10 MINUTES · COOK TIME: 10 MINUTES

Consider adding a bun for more carbohydrates in this healthy version of the Southern classic. Most buns are 2 to 3 ounces, or the equivalent of 30 to 45 grams of carbohydrate. You'll enjoy the flavors of the tasty seasoning on the seafood and spicy Remoulade on top.

1 cup whole-wheat bread crumbs

2 teaspoons sea salt

1 teaspoon dried oregano

¼ teaspoon cayenne (or to taste)

½ cup whole-wheat flour

2 large eggs

1 pound sea scallops

4 large lettuce leaves, for serving

1 recipe Remoulade (page 131), for serving

PER SERVING Calories: 447; Total Fat: 20g; Saturated Fat: 3g; Sodium: 1349mg; Carbohydrates: 37g; Fiber: 2g; Protein: 28g

1. Preheat the oven to 450°F.

2. In a medium bowl, whisk together the bread crumbs, salt, oregano, and cayenne until well combined.

3. Put the flour in a separate bowl.

4. In a small bowl, beat the eggs well.

5. Dip the scallops in the flour and pat off any excess. Dip them in the eggs, and then into the bread crumb mixture. Place on a rimmed baking sheet.

6. Bake until the breading is browned, 8 to 10 minutes.

7. Spoon the scallops into the lettuce leaves. Serve topped with the Remoulade.

STORAGE NOTE: Store the cooked scallops separately from the sauce and the lettuce for up to 3 days in the refrigerator.

RECIPE TIP: You can avoid the bread crumbs and simply dip the scallops in the eggs and flour. This reduces the carbohydrate grams by as much as 18 grams per serving. When adjusting recipes, be sure to rethink the carbohydrate component of the entire meal.

TERIYAKI SALMON

≤10 · DAIRY-FREE · NUT-FREE

SERVES 4 · PREP TIME: 5 MINUTES · COOK TIME: 4 MINUTES

Teriyaki has a sweet, salty flavor that pairs nicely with the sweet flavor of salmon. To make this gluten-free, you can use gluten-free soy sauce. If you can't find rice vinegar, regular white vinegar is an acceptable substitute.

⅓ cup pineapple juice
⅓ cup reduced-sodium soy sauce
¼ cup water
2 tablespoons rice vinegar
1 tablespoon honey
1 garlic clove, minced
1 teaspoon peeled and grated fresh ginger
Pinch red pepper flakes
1 pound salmon fillet, cut into 4 pieces

PER SERVING Calories: 202; Total Fat: 7g; Saturated Fat: 1g; Sodium: 752mg; Carbohydrates: 9g; Fiber: <1g; Protein: 24g

1. Preheat the oven broiler on high.

2. In a small bowl, whisk together the pineapple juice, soy sauce, water, vinegar, honey, garlic, ginger, and red pepper flakes.

3. Place the salmon pieces flesh-side down in the mixture for 5 minutes.

4. Place the salmon on a rimmed baking sheet, flesh-side up. Gently brush with any leftover sauce.

5. Broil until the salmon is opaque, 3 to 5 minutes.

STORAGE NOTE: Store in the refrigerator for up to 3 days.

RECIPE TIP: This is a very-low-carb recipe, even with the honey and pineapple juice. You can increase the carbs by serving it with Asian Chicken Slaw (page 70), making the slaw but omitting the chicken, or serve with a side of steamed veggies.

EASY TUNA PATTIES

DAIRY-FREE · NUT-FREE

SERVES 4 · PREP TIME: 5 MINUTES, PLUS 10 MINUTES TO CHILL · COOK TIME: 10 MINUTES

By themselves, these patties are low in carbs, even with the inclusion of whole-wheat bread crumbs. You can enjoy them with a knife and fork, or if you have a few carbs to spare, put them on slices of whole-grain toast as an open-faced sandwich.

1 pound canned tuna, drained

1 cup whole-wheat bread crumbs

2 large eggs, beaten

½ onion, grated

1 tablespoon chopped fresh dill

Juice and zest of 1 lemon

3 tablespoons extra-virgin olive oil

½ cup tartar sauce, for serving

PER SERVING Calories: 530; Total Fat: 34g; Saturated Fat: 5g; Sodium: 674mg; Carbohydrates: 18g; Fiber: 2g; Protein: 35g

1. In a large bowl, combine the tuna, bread crumbs, eggs, onion, dill, and lemon juice and zest. Form the mixture into 4 patties and chill for 10 minutes.

2. In a large nonstick skillet over medium-high heat, heat the olive oil until it shimmers. Add the patties and cook until browned on both sides, 4 to 5 minutes per side.

3. Serve topped with the tartar sauce.

STORAGE NOTE: Store in the refrigerator for up to 3 days.

RECIPE TIP: Making this an open-faced sandwich with one slice of whole-wheat bread adds an estimated 15 grams of carbs. You can also serve this with a simple side salad of non-starchy veggies and a low-sugar vinaigrette for a complete meal.

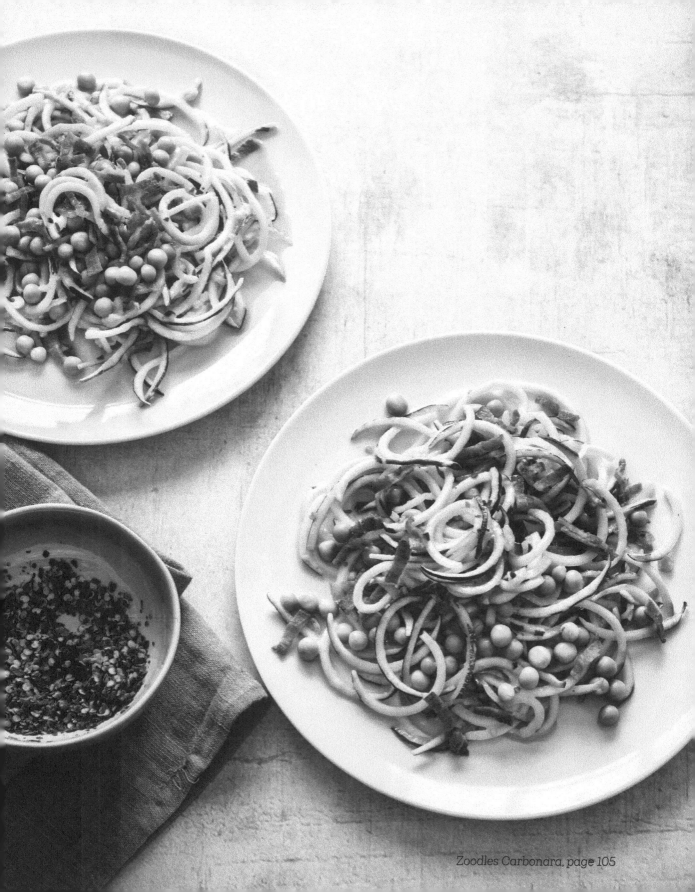

Zoodles Carbonara, page 105

Poultry and Meat Mains

TURKEY SCALOPPINI

≤15 · NUT-FREE · ONE-POT

SERVES 4 · PREP TIME: 10 MINUTES · COOK TIME: 20 MINUTES

Since the turkey breast is pounded flat, it cooks in a snap, and you'll finish it off with a flavorful and fast pan sauce. To pound the turkey breast, cut it into ½-inch-thick slices, and then place the slices between two sheets of plastic wrap. Use a mallet or something heavy with a flat bottom to pound it to ¼-inch thickness.

½ cup whole-wheat flour

½ teaspoon sea salt

¼ teaspoon freshly ground black pepper

3 tablespoons extra-virgin olive oil

12 ounces turkey breast, cut into ½-inch-thick cutlets and pounded flat (see headnote)

1 garlic clove, minced

½ cup dry white wine

2 tablespoons chopped fresh rosemary

1 cup low-sodium chicken broth

2 tablespoons salted butter, very cold, cut into small pieces

PER SERVING Calories: 344; Total Fat: 20g; Saturated Fat: 7g; Sodium: 266mg; Carbohydrates: 15g; Fiber: 2g; Protein: 24g

1. Preheat the oven to 200°F. Line a baking sheet with parchment paper.

2. In a medium bowl, whisk together the flour, salt, and pepper.

3. In a large skillet over medium-high heat, heat the olive oil until it shimmers.

4. Working in batches with one or two pieces of turkey at a time (depending on how much room you have in the pan), dredge the turkey cutlets in the flour and pat off any excess. Cook in the hot oil until the turkey is cooked through, about 3 minutes per side. Add more oil if needed.

5. Place the cooked cutlets on the lined baking sheet and keep them warm in the oven while you cook the remaining turkey and make the pan sauce.

6. Once all the turkey is cooked and warming in the oven, add the garlic to the pan and cook, stirring constantly, for 30 seconds. Add the wine and use the side of a spoon to scrape any browned bits off the bottom of the pan. Simmer, stirring, for 1 minute. Add the rosemary and chicken broth. Simmer, stirring, until it thickens, 1 to 2 minutes more.

7. Whisk in the cold butter, one piece at a time, until incorporated. Return the turkey cutlets to the sauce and turn once to coat.

Serve with any remaining sauce spooned over the top.

STORAGE NOTE: If not eating right away, you can store the cooked cutlets and extra sauce separately in the refrigerator for up to 3 days.

RECIPE TIP: Serve the turkey and sauce over zucchini noodles—each cup has about 7 grams of carbs and 2 grams of fiber—and add a steamed veggie or side salad.

GROUND TURKEY TACO SKILLET

GLUTEN-FREE · NUT-FREE · ONE-POT

SERVES 4 · PREP TIME: 10 MINUTES · COOK TIME: 20 MINUTES

Using prepared salsa is a simple way to add flavor to ground turkey. This is a delicious Southwestern one-pot meal that's pretty versatile, too. You can use leftovers as taco meat or serve them over a bed of lettuce and other greens for a tasty taco salad. Top with your favorite Southwestern toppings, such as sour cream or diced avocados.

3 tablespoons extra-virgin olive oil

1 pound ground turkey

1 onion, chopped

1 green bell pepper, seeded and chopped

½ teaspoon sea salt

1 small head cauliflower, grated

1 cup corn kernels

½ cup prepared salsa

1 cup shredded pepper Jack cheese

PER SERVING Calories: 448; Total Fat: 30g; Saturated Fat: 10g; Sodium: 649mg; Carbohydrates: 18g; Fiber: 4g; Protein: 30g

1. In a large nonstick skillet over medium-high heat, heat the olive oil until it shimmers.

2. Add the turkey. Cook, crumbling with a spoon, until browned, about 5 minutes.

3. Add the onion, bell pepper, and salt. Cook, stirring occasionally, until the vegetables soften, 4 to 5 minutes.

4. Add the cauliflower, corn, and salsa. Cook, stirring, until the cauliflower rice softens, about 3 minutes more.

5. Sprinkle with the cheese. Reduce heat to low, cover, and allow the cheese to melt, 2 or 3 minutes.

STORAGE NOTE: Refrigerate in a sealed container for up to 3 days, or freeze for up to 6 months.

RECIPE TIP: Using cauliflower in place of rice makes this a fairly low-carb dinner. If you need a few extra grams of carbs, replace the cauliflower with 1 cup of cooked brown rice. It is estimated that 1 cup cooked rice has 45 grams of carbs, but check the nutrition facts label to be sure.

TURKEY MEATLOAF MEATBALLS

NUT-FREE

SERVES 4 · PREP TIME: 10 MINUTES · COOK TIME: 20 MINUTES

Meatloaf takes a while to cook in the oven. However, you can get all the flavor of meatloaf in about a third of the cooking time by turning the mixture into meatballs. So the next time you crave meatloaf **now**, make it into meatballs and it will be on the table in 30 minutes or less. The bread crumbs and milk form a binder that holds the meatballs together and keeps them moist and tender.

¼ **cup tomato paste**

1 **tablespoon honey**

1 **tablespoon Worcestershire sauce**

½ **cup milk**

½ **cup whole-wheat bread crumbs**

1 **pound ground turkey**

1 **onion, grated**

1 **tablespoon Dijon mustard**

1 **teaspoon dried thyme**

½ **teaspoon sea salt**

PER SERVING Calories: 285; Total Fat: 11g; Saturated Fat: 3g; Sodium: 465mg; Carbohydrates: 22g; Fiber: 2g; Protein: 24g

1. Preheat the oven to 375°F. Line a rimmed baking sheet with parchment paper.

2. In a small saucepan on medium-low heat, whisk together the tomato paste, honey, and Worcestershire sauce. Bring to a simmer and then remove from the heat.

3. In a large bowl, combine the milk and bread crumbs. Let rest for 5 minutes.

4. Add the ground turkey, onion, mustard, thyme, and salt. Using your hands, mix well without overmixing.

(Continued)

5. Form into 1-inch meatballs and place on the prepared baking sheet. Brush the tops with the tomato paste mixture.

6. Bake until the meatballs reach 165°F internally, about 15 minutes.

STORAGE NOTE: Freeze in single-serving containers or resealable bags for up to 6 months, or refrigerate for up to 3 days.

RECIPE TIP: The traditional accompaniment to meatloaf is mashed potatoes. Consider adding higher-fiber starches, such as cooked quinoa, wild rice, or half of a sweet potato. Remember as you add carbohydrates to use your measuring cups or digital scale to understand how much is added; you will need to dose on total carbs in the meal. An average ⅓- to ½-cup serving of starchy vegetables or 1 ounce of whole-grain breads will add 15 grams of carbs.

BAKED CHICKEN TENDERS

DAIRY-FREE

SERVES 4 · PREP TIME: 10 MINUTES · COOK TIME: 15 MINUTES

Cutting chicken into ½-inch-thick pieces and pounding it slightly so that the pieces are the same thickness helps it cook evenly. You can use either thigh meat or breast meat; both cuts have no carbohydrates and similar amounts of protein. However, the thigh is higher in fat. Serve these with any of the sauces in chapter 9, such as Remoulade (page 131), Peanut Sauce (page 133), or Chimichurri (page 129), with a side salad or Garlic Kale Chips (page 50).

1 cup whole-wheat bread crumbs

1 tablespoon dried thyme

1 teaspoon garlic powder

1 teaspoon paprika

½ teaspoon sea salt

3 large eggs, beaten

1 tablespoon Dijon mustard

1 pound chicken, cut into ½-inch-thick pieces and pounded to even thickness

STORAGE NOTE: Refrigerate in a sealed container for up to 3 days, or freeze for up to 6 months. Reheat in a 375°F oven for about 15 minutes.

PER SERVING Calories: 276; Total Fat: 6g; Saturated Fat: 2g; Sodium: 487mg; Carbohydrates: 17g; Fiber: 3g; Protein: 34g

1. Preheat the oven to 375°F. Line a rimmed baking sheet with parchment paper.

2. In a medium bowl, whisk together the bread crumbs, thyme, garlic powder, paprika, and salt.

3. In another bowl, whisk together the eggs and mustard.

4. Dip each piece of chicken in the egg mixture and then in the bread crumb mixture. Place on the prepared baking sheet.

5. Bake until the chicken reaches an internal temperature of 165°F and the bread crumbs are golden, about 15 minutes.

RECIPE TIP: Serve these tenders on a bed of greens as a salad, or enjoy each serving with 1 cup cooked sweet potato, which adds an estimated 30 grams of carbohydrates. Use a resource guide and a digital scale when adding potato.

CHICKEN WITH
LEMON CAPER PAN SAUCE

≤10 · GLUTEN-FREE · NUT-FREE · ONE-POT

SERVES 4 · PREP TIME: 10 MINUTES · COOK TIME: 15 MINUTES

You can use either skinless boneless breasts or thighs here. Pound them slightly between two pieces of plastic wrap to an even thickness so the chicken cooks evenly. The lemon caper sauce adds tasty elements of salt and acid to the sweet flavor of the chicken.

3 tablespoons extra-virgin olive oil

4 chicken breast halves or thighs, pounded slightly to even thickness

½ teaspoon sea salt

⅛ teaspoon freshly ground black pepper

¼ cup freshly squeezed lemon juice

¼ cup dry white wine

2 tablespoons capers, rinsed

2 tablespoons salted butter, very cold, cut into pieces

PER SERVING Calories: 281; Total Fat: 17g; Saturated Fat: 5g; Sodium: 386mg; Carbohydrates: 2g; Fiber: <1g; Protein: 26g

1. In a large skillet over medium-high heat, heat the olive oil until it shimmers.

2. Season the chicken with the salt and pepper. Add it to the hot oil and cook until opaque with an internal temperature of 165°F, about 5 minutes per side. Transfer the chicken to a plate and tent loosely with foil to keep warm. Keep the pan on the heat.

3. Add the lemon juice and wine to the pan, using the side of a spoon to scrape any browned bits from the bottom of the pan. Add the capers. Simmer until the liquid is reduced by half, about 3 minutes. Reduce the heat to low.

The Type 1 Diabetes Cookbook

4. Whisk in the butter, one piece at a time, until incorporated.

5. Return the chicken to the pan, turning once to coat with the sauce. Serve with additional sauce spooned over the top.

STORAGE NOTE: Refrigerate for up to 3 days, storing the sauce separately from the chicken.

RECIPE TIP: Since this is a simple chicken with a sauce, it is very low in carbohydrates. Add more carbs with your sides. You can serve a starch, such as ⅓ cup of cooked brown rice, wild rice, or barley, and spoon the pan sauce over the top. The extra carbs add approximately 15 grams per ½ cup. For only 5 grams of carbohydrates, sauté spinach in olive oil and squeeze a little lemon over the top.

CHICKEN SATAY STIR-FRY

DAIRY-FREE · ONE-POT

SERVES 4 · PREP TIME: 10 MINUTES · COOK TIME: 15 MINUTES

The trick to this easy, Thai-inspired stir-fry is the tasty Peanut Sauce, which serves as the binding sauce of the stir-fry and flavors all the other ingredients. This recipe calls for riced cauliflower. While you can sometimes buy this form of cauliflower at the grocery store, it's so easy to make on your own by grating cauliflower on a box grater or pulsing it in a food processor until it resembles rice.

3 tablespoons extra-virgin olive oil

1 pound chicken breasts or thighs, cut into ¾-inch pieces

½ teaspoon sea salt

2 cups broccoli florets

1 red bell pepper, seeded and chopped

6 scallions, green and white parts, sliced on the bias (cut diagonally into thin slices)

1 head cauliflower, riced

Peanut Sauce (page 133)

STORAGE NOTE: This will store in the refrigerator for up to 3 days. It doesn't freeze well.

PER SERVING Calories: 381; Total Fat: 20g; Saturated Fat: 4g; Sodium: 396mg; Carbohydrates: 19g; Fiber: 5g; Protein: 33g

1. In a large skillet over medium-high heat, heat the olive oil until it shimmers.

2. Season the chicken with the salt. Add the chicken to the oil and cook, stirring occasionally, until opaque, about 5 minutes. Remove the chicken from the oil with a slotted spoon and set it aside on a plate. Return the pan to the heat.

3. Add the broccoli, bell pepper, and scallions. Cook, stirring, until the vegetables are crisp-tender, 3 to 5 minutes. Add the cauliflower and cook for 3 minutes more.

4. Return the chicken to the skillet. Stir in the Peanut Sauce. Bring to a simmer and reduce heat to medium-low. Simmer to heat through, about 2 minutes more.

RECIPE TIP: For a few more grams of carbs and a more traditional Asian dish, you can replace the cauliflower with 1 cup of cooked brown rice, which will add 45 grams of carbs, or about 11 grams per serving. You can also add more veggies, such as mushrooms or kale. When adding raw non-starchy vegetables, count an extra 5 grams of carbohydrate per cup.

ASIAN CHICKEN STIR-FRY

≤15 · DAIRY-FREE · NUT-FREE

SERVES 4 · PREP TIME: 10 MINUTES · COOK TIME: 10 MINUTES

This recipe focuses on traditional Asian flavors, such as ginger, lime, sesame oil, and garlic. It's easy to customize this stir-fry with your favorite non-starchy vegetables, which will add very few carbs.

3 tablespoons extra-virgin olive oil

1 pound chicken breasts or thighs, cut into ¾-inch pieces

2 cups edamame or pea pods

3 garlic cloves, chopped

1 tablespoon peeled and grated fresh ginger

2 tablespoons reduced-sodium soy sauce

Juice of 2 limes

1 teaspoon sesame oil

2 teaspoons toasted sesame seeds

1 tablespoon chopped fresh cilantro

PER SERVING Calories: 331; Total Fat: 17g; Saturated Fat: 2g; Sodium: 342mg; Carbohydrates: 11g; Fiber: 5g; Protein: 31g

1. In a large skillet over medium-high heat, heat the olive oil until it shimmers. Add the chicken to the oil and cook, stirring occasionally, until opaque, about 5 minutes. Add the edamame and cook, stirring occasionally, until crisp-tender, 3 to 5 minutes. Add the garlic and ginger and cook, stirring constantly, for 30 seconds.

2. In a small bowl, whisk together the soy sauce, lime juice, and sesame oil. Add the sauce mixture to the pan. Bring to a simmer, stirring, and cook for 2 minutes.

3. Remove from heat and garnish with the sesame seeds and cilantro.

STORAGE NOTE: This will store in the refrigerator for up to 3 days. It doesn't freeze well.

RECIPE TIP: Pea pods are a lower-carbohydrate alternative to edamame. Be sure to subtract about 10 grams of carbs if you are replacing the edamame with pea pods.

ORANGE CHICKEN

≤10 · DAIRY-FREE · GLUTEN-FREE · NUT-FREE

SERVES 4 · PREP TIME: 10 MINUTES · COOK TIME: 10 MINUTES

Sweet, acidic, and slightly spicy, orange chicken is a perennial favorite for Asian takeout. It's usually pretty high in carbs, however, due to the sugar in the sauce and the heavy breading on the chicken. This version preserves the flavors but removes the breading and sugar, so you can add more veggies on the side instead.

3 tablespoons extra-virgin olive oil

1 pound chicken breasts or thighs, cut into ¾-inch pieces

1 teaspoon peeled and grated fresh ginger

2 garlic cloves, minced

1 tablespoon honey

Juice and zest of 1 orange

1 teaspoon cornstarch

½ teaspoon sriracha (or to taste)

Sesame seeds (optional, for garnish)

Thinly sliced scallion (optional, for garnish)

PER SERVING Calories: 245; Total Fat: 12g; Saturated Fat: 2g; Sodium: 75mg; Carbohydrates: 9g; Fiber: <1g; Protein: 26g

1. In a large skillet over medium-high heat, heat the olive oil until it shimmers. Add the chicken to the oil and cook, stirring occasionally, until opaque, about 5 minutes. Add the ginger and garlic and cook, stirring constantly, for 30 seconds.

2. In a small bowl, whisk together the honey, orange juice and zest, cornstarch, and sriracha. Add the sauce mixture to the chicken and cook, stirring, until the sauce thickens, about 2 minutes.

3. Serve garnished with sesame seeds and sliced scallions, if desired.

STORAGE NOTE: Refrigerate in a sealed container for up to 3 days, or freeze for up to 6 months.

RECIPE TIP: With the low carb counts in this recipe, you can add red onions or red bell peppers to the stir-fry. Cook the vegetables after the chicken is cooked. It's best to remove the chicken, cook the vegetables in the sauce, and then return the cooked chicken to the pan. Serve over cauliflower rice.

ZOODLES CARBONARA

≤15 · GLUTEN-FREE · NUT-FREE · ONE-POT

SERVES 4 · PREP TIME: 10 MINUTES · COOK TIME: 25 MINUTES

Carbonara is a simple bacon-and-egg sauce that is normally served over pasta, but it's delicious on spiralized zucchini, too. Delicious in its simplicity, it's fast and easy to make. Choose a nice pepper bacon for a sharper bite or pancetta for a lighter flavor, or pick your favorite artisanal bacon to accentuate this delicious "pasta" dish.

6 slices bacon, cut into pieces

1 red onion, finely chopped

3 zucchini, cut into noodles

1 cup peas

½ teaspoon sea salt

3 garlic cloves, minced

3 large eggs, beaten

1 tablespoon heavy cream

Pinch red pepper flakes

½ cup grated Parmesan cheese (optional, for garnish)

STORAGE NOTE: This doesn't keep well. You can refrigerate leftovers, but they won't be as good upon reheating.

PER SERVING Calories: 326; Total Fat: 24g; Saturated Fat: 8g; Sodium: 555mg; Carbohydrates: 15g; Fiber: 4g; Protein: 14g

1. In a large skillet over medium-high heat, cook the bacon until browned, about 5 minutes. With a slotted spoon, transfer the bacon to a plate.

2. Add the onion to the bacon fat in the pan and cook, stirring, until soft, 3 to 5 minutes. Add the zucchini, peas, and salt. Cook, stirring, until the zucchini softens, about 3 minutes. Add the garlic and cook, stirring constantly, for 5 minutes.

3. In a small bowl, whisk together the eggs, cream, and red pepper flakes. Add to the vegetables.

4. Remove the pan from the stove top and stir for 3 minutes, allowing the heat of the pan to cook the eggs without setting them.

5. Return the bacon to the pan and stir to mix.

6. Serve topped with Parmesan cheese, if desired.

RECIPE TIP: The peas in this recipe add protein and some carbs. If you need a slightly higher-carb version, you can add more peas. For every additional ½ cup of peas, add 15 grams of carbohydrate.

PORK AND APPLE SKILLET

DAIRY-FREE · GLUTEN-FREE · NUT-FREE · ONE-POT

SERVES 4 · PREP TIME: 10 MINUTES · COOK TIME: 20 MINUTES

Pork and apples are a great combination, particularly in the fall, when apples are in season. Choose a tart-sweet apple, such as Honeycrisp, Granny Smith, or Cripps pink. Save time by using coleslaw mix instead of shredding a head of cabbage.

1 pound ground pork

1 red onion, thinly sliced

2 apples, peeled, cored, and thinly sliced

2 cups shredded cabbage

1 teaspoon dried thyme

2 garlic cloves, minced

¼ cup apple cider vinegar

1 tablespoon Dijon mustard

½ teaspoon sea salt

⅛ teaspoon freshly ground black pepper

STORAGE NOTE: Refrigerate in a sealed container for up to 3 days, or freeze for up to 6 months.

PER SERVING Calories: 364; Total Fat: 24g; Saturated Fat: 9g; Sodium: 260mg; Carbohydrates: 19g; Fiber: 4g; Protein: 20g

1. In a large skillet over medium-high heat, cook the ground pork, crumbling it with a spoon, until browned, about 5 minutes. Use a slotted spoon to transfer the pork to a plate.

2. Add the onion, apples, cabbage, and thyme to the fat in the pan. Cook, stirring occasionally, until the vegetables are soft, about 5 minutes.

3. Add the garlic and cook, stirring constantly, for 5 minutes.

4. Return the pork to the pan.

5. In a small bowl, whisk together the vinegar, mustard, salt, and pepper. Add to the pan. Bring to a simmer. Cook, stirring, until the sauce thickens, about 2 minutes.

RECIPE TIP: Replace the ground pork with a few pounds of country-style pork ribs, toss all the uncooked ingredients into a slow cooker, and cook on low for 8 hours. You'll be rewarded with a flavorful crockpot dinner that takes very little prep work. This dish is delicious served with sautéed Swiss chard, which is a green leafy vegetable that adds few carbs and is an excellent source of calcium.

VEGETABLE BEEF SOUP

DAIRY-FREE · GLUTEN-FREE · NUT-FREE · ONE-POT

SERVES 4 · PREP TIME: 10 MINUTES · COOK TIME: 15 MINUTES

Using ground beef and onions as your soup base means this soup cooks very quickly. It's a great soup to make in large batches, because it freezes and travels well and reheats easily on the stove top or in the microwave. You can add different non-starchy veggies depending on your taste. To save even more time, use frozen vegetables.

1 pound ground beef

1 onion, chopped

2 celery stalks, chopped

1 carrot, chopped

1 teaspoon dried rosemary

6 cups low-sodium beef or chicken broth

½ teaspoon sea salt

⅛ teaspoon freshly ground black pepper

2 cups peas

PER SERVING Calories: 355; Total Fat: 17g; Saturated Fat: 7g; Sodium: 362mg; Carbohydrates:18g; Fiber: 5g; Protein: 34g

1. In a large pot over medium-high heat, cook the ground beef, crumbling with the side of a spoon, until browned, about 5 minutes.

2. Add the onion, celery, carrot, and rosemary. Cook, stirring occasionally, until the vegetables start to soften, about 5 minutes.

3. Add the broth, salt, pepper, and peas. Bring to a simmer. Reduce the heat and simmer, stirring, until warmed through, about 5 minutes more.

STORAGE NOTE: Refrigerate in a sealed container for up to 3 days, or freeze for up to 6 months.

RECIPE TIP: To add some carbs, you can add cooked barley, which adds heartiness to the soup. Add the cooked barley when you add the peas. Use a resource guide for adding extra carbohydrates, or use the general guideline of ⅓ cup cooked barley equaling 15 grams carbs.

OPEN-FACED PUB-STYLE BISON BURGERS

NUT-FREE

SERVES 4 · PREP TIME: 10 MINUTES · COOK TIME: 15 MINUTES

If you can't find ground bison or buffalo, feel free to substitute ground beef. These burgers are a real treat, with piquant blue cheese, sweet onions, and the slightly gamy flavor of the bison. Add the creamy and tangy Pub Sauce, and it makes the perfect burger.

2 tablespoons extra-virgin olive oil

1 onion, thinly sliced

1 pound ground bison

1 teaspoon sea salt, divided

1 cup blue cheese crumbles

4 slices sourdough bread

1 garlic clove, halved

Pub Sauce (page 132)

PER SERVING Calories: 390; Total Fat: 23g; Saturated Fat: 4g; Sodium: 793mg; Carbohydrates: 22g; Fiber: 1g; Protein: 27g

1. In a large skillet over medium-high heat, heat the olive oil until it shimmers. Add the onion. Cook, stirring, until it begins to brown, about 5 minutes.

2. Set the onion aside, and wipe out the skillet with a paper towel and return it to the stove at medium-high heat. Season the bison with the salt and form it into 4 patties. Brown the patties in the hot skillet until they reach an internal temperature of 140°F, about 5 minutes per side.

3. Sprinkle the blue cheese over the tops of the burgers and remove the skillet from the heat. Cover the skillet and allow the cheese to melt.

4. Meanwhile, toast the bread and then rub the garlic halves over the pieces of toast to flavor them.

5. To assemble, put a piece of toast on a plate. Top with onion slices, place a burger patty on top, and then spoon the sauce over the patty.

STORAGE NOTE: Store the sauce, bread, onion, and patties separately. Refrigerate sauce, patties, and onion for up to 3 days.

RECIPE TIP: When using sourdough bread, bring out your digital scale. Remember, 1 ounce of most bread products adds 15 grams of carbohydrates. Adjust insulin accordingly and enjoy the burger! If you are avoiding bread, you can serve the burger topped with onion slices and sauce.

BROCCOLI BEEF STIR-FRY

≤10 · DAIRY-FREE · NUT-FREE

SERVES 4 · PREP TIME: 10 MINUTES · COOK TIME: 15 MINUTES

Stir-fries are fast, particularly when you cut the meat thinly. To make easy work of cutting the meat into thin strips, wrap it in plastic and freeze it for about 10 minutes to firm the meat up before slicing. You can also use frozen stir-fry veggies for an even quicker meal.

2 tablespoons extra-virgin olive oil

1 pound sirloin steak, cut into ¼-inch-thick strips

2 cups broccoli florets

1 garlic clove, minced

1 teaspoon peeled and grated fresh ginger

2 tablespoons reduced-sodium soy sauce

¼ cup beef broth

½ teaspoon Chinese hot mustard

Pinch red pepper flakes

STORAGE NOTE: Refrigerate in a sealed container for up to 3 days, or freeze for up to 6 months.

PER SERVING Calories: 227; Total Fat: 11g; Saturated Fat: 2g; Sodium: 375mg; Carbohydrates: 5g; Fiber: 1g; Protein: 27g

1. In a large skillet over medium-high heat, heat the olive oil until it shimmers. Add the beef. Cook, stirring, until it browns, 3 to 5 minutes. With a slotted spoon, remove the beef from the oil and set it aside on a plate.

2. Add the broccoli to the oil. Cook, stirring, until it is crisp-tender, about 4 minutes.

3. Add the garlic and ginger and cook, stirring constantly, for 30 seconds.

4. Return the beef to the pan, along with any juices that have collected.

5. In a small bowl, whisk together the soy sauce, broth, mustard, and red pepper flakes.

6. Add the soy sauce mixture to the skillet and cook, stirring, until everything warms through, about 3 minutes.

RECIPE TIP: Check your blood sugars to adjust insulin for low-carb meals. You can add more veggies to the stir-fry without significantly changing the carb counts. Onions and chopped red bell peppers work well with this recipe.

BEEF AND PEPPER FAJITA BOWLS

≤15 · DAIRY-FREE · NUT-FREE · ONE-POT

SERVES 4 · PREP TIME: 10 MINUTES · COOK TIME: 15 MINUTES

You won't even miss the tortillas when you make these delicious fajita bowls. If desired, serve topped with cheese, sour cream, or even guacamole (see page 54). These fajita bowls are flavorful and aromatic, and they make a popular family meal as an alternative to tacos on taco night.

4 tablespoons extra-virgin olive oil, divided

1 head cauliflower, riced

1 pound sirloin steak, cut into ¼-inch-thick strips

1 red bell pepper, seeded and sliced

1 onion, thinly sliced

2 garlic cloves, minced

Juice of 2 limes

1 teaspoon chili powder

PER SERVING Calories: 310; Total Fat: 18g; Saturated Fat: 3g; Sodium: 93mg; Carbohydrates: 13g; Fiber: 3g; Protein: 27g

1. In a large skillet over medium-high heat, heat 2 tablespoons of olive oil until it shimmers. Add the cauliflower. Cook, stirring occasionally, until it softens, about 3 minutes. Set aside.

2. Wipe out the skillet with a paper towel. Add the remaining 2 tablespoons of oil to the skillet, and heat it on medium-high until it shimmers. Add the steak and cook, stirring occasionally, until it browns, about 3 minutes. Use a slotted spoon to remove the steak from the oil in the pan and set aside.

3. Add the bell pepper and onion to the pan. Cook, stirring occasionally, until they start to brown, about 5 minutes.

(Continued)

4. Add the garlic and cook, stirring constantly, for 30 seconds.

5. Return the beef along with any juices that have collected and the cauliflower to the pan. Add the lime juice and chili powder. Cook, stirring, until everything is warmed through, 2 to 3 minutes.

STORAGE NOTE: Refrigerate in a sealed container for up to 3 days, or freeze for up to 6 months.

RECIPE TIP: The carbs in this dish are right in the sweet spot. However, if you have a workout coming up and could use a few extra carbs, you can add a 6-inch low-carb tortilla on the side, which adds 12 grams of carbs with 8 grams of fiber per tortilla.

LAMB KOFTA MEATBALLS WITH CUCUMBER QUICK-PICKLED SALAD

≤10 · DAIRY-FREE · GLUTEN-FREE · NUT-FREE

SERVES 4 · PREP TIME: 10 MINUTES · COOK TIME: 15 MINUTES

With fragrant spices and a cool cucumber and red onion salad, this main dish offers the perfect blend of flavors and aromas. Mix the salad first so the flavors have time to blend, and then make the meatballs, baking them in the oven for about 15 minutes while the salad pickles slightly.

¼ cup red wine vinegar

Pinch red pepper flakes

1 teaspoon sea salt, divided

2 cucumbers, peeled and chopped

½ red onion, finely chopped

1 pound ground lamb

2 teaspoons ground coriander

1 teaspoon ground cumin

3 garlic cloves, minced

1 tablespoon fresh mint, chopped

STORAGE NOTE: Store the salad and lamb separately in the refrigerator for up to 3 days. The meatballs can be frozen for up to 6 months. The salad doesn't freeze well.

PER SERVING Calories: 345; Total Fat: 27g; Saturated Fat: 12g; Sodium: 362mg; Carbohydrates: 7g; Fiber: 1g; Protein: 20g

1. Preheat the oven to 375°F. Line a rimmed baking sheet with parchment paper.

2. In a medium bowl, whisk together the vinegar, red pepper flakes, and ½ teaspoon of salt. Add the cucumbers and onion and toss to combine. Set aside.

3. In a large bowl, mix the lamb, coriander, cumin, garlic, mint, and remaining ½ teaspoon of salt. Form the mixture into 1-inch meatballs and place them on the prepared baking sheet.

4. Bake until the lamb reaches 140°F internally, about 15 minutes.

5. Serve with the salad on the side.

RECIPE TIP: Try this with whole-wheat couscous, which adds about 12 grams of carbs and 2 grams of fiber per ¼-cup cooked serving. Toss the couscous with some olive oil, red wine vinegar, and freshly chopped mint and oregano for a simple side that pairs perfectly with this dinner. Take out your measuring cups when you eat couscous and other cooked grains to be sure you are accurately noting portions.

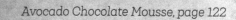
Avocado Chocolate Mousse, page 122

CHAPTER EIGHT

Desserts

ICE CREAM WITH WARM STRAWBERRY RHUBARB SAUCE

GLUTEN-FREE · NUT-FREE · ONE-POT · VEGETARIAN

SERVES 4 · PREP TIME: 10 MINUTES · COOK TIME: 15 MINUTES

Strawberries are a good source of soluble fiber, and rhubarb is a healthy vegetable with an estimated 6 grams carbohydrates per cup. Together, they deliver a sweet-tart flavor that's irresistible, especially if you pair it with sugar-free ice cream. While this recipe is low in carbs for a dessert, it's still important to consider the carbohydrate grams and bolus insulin when eating this dessert.

1 cup sliced strawberries

1 cup chopped rhubarb

2 tablespoons water

1 tablespoon honey

½ teaspoon cinnamon

4 (¼-cup) scoops sugar-free vanilla ice cream

PER SERVING Calories: 86; Total Fat: 2g; Saturated Fat: 1g; Sodium: 37mg; Carbohydrates: 16g; Fiber: 3g; Protein: 3g

1. In a medium pot, combine the strawberries, rhubarb, water, honey, and cinnamon. Bring to a simmer on medium heat, stirring. Reduce the heat to medium-low. Simmer, stirring frequently, until the rhubarb is soft, about 15 minutes. Allow to cool slightly.

2. Place 1 scoop of ice cream into each of 4 bowls. Spoon the sauce over the ice cream.

STORAGE NOTE: The sauce will store well refrigerated for up to 5 days.

RECIPE TIP: Omitting the ice cream reduces carb counts to 9 grams per serving. Replacing the ice cream with plain Greek yogurt decreases carbs to about 21 grams per serving.

BLACKBERRY YOGURT ICE POPS

≤10 · GLUTEN-FREE · NUT-FREE · VEGETARIAN

SERVES 4 · PREP TIME: 10 MINUTES, PLUS 6 HOURS TO FREEZE · COOK TIME: NONE

Children and adults love this refreshing dessert that provides an alternative to high-fat yogurts, which are often topped with high-sugar candies. If you don't have ice pop molds, you can make these using paper cups. Pour the mixture into four cups (or six if you have smaller cups), cover them with foil, insert a stick through the foil to hold it in place, and then freeze. To serve, peel away the paper cups.

12 ounces plain Greek yogurt

1 cup blackberries

Pinch nutmeg

¼ cup milk

2 (1-gram) packets stevia

PER SERVING Calories: 75; Total Fat: 6g; Saturated Fat: 0g; Sodium: 7mg; Carbohydrates: 9g; Fiber: 2g; Protein: 9g

1. In a blender, combine all of the ingredients. Blend until smooth.

2. Pour the mixture into 4 ice pop molds. Freeze for 6 hours before serving.

STORAGE NOTE: You can keep these in the freezer for up to 6 months.

RECIPE TIP: Replace the Greek yogurt with 2 cups of full-fat canned coconut milk and omit the milk. This reduces carbs to 10 grams per serving and provides 5 grams of fiber (and makes it dairy-free). Remember to take insulin with snacks.

COFFEE AND CREAM POPS

≤10 · DAIRY-FREE · GLUTEN-FREE · NUT-FREE · VEGAN

SERVES 4 · PREP TIME: 10 MINUTES, PLUS 6 HOURS TO FREEZE · COOK TIME: 5 MINUTES

If you love the flavor of coffee, you'll enjoy this delicious dessert. It's like a sweetened latte as an ice pop. This version uses creamy coconut milk, but you could also use half-and-half or an unsweetened nut milk (such as almond milk). It will alter the texture and be slightly less creamy, but still delicious. Almond milk is the better alternative, especially if you do not want any saturated fats.

2 teaspoons espresso powder (or to taste)
2 cups canned coconut milk
½ teaspoon vanilla extract
½ teaspoon cinnamon
3 (1-gram) packets stevia

PER SERVING Calories: 225; Total Fat: 24g; Saturated Fat: 21g; Sodium: 15mg; Carbohydrates: 7g; Fiber: 3g; Protein: 2g

1. In a medium saucepan over medium-low heat, heat all of the ingredients, stirring constantly, until the espresso powder is completely dissolved, about 5 minutes.

2. Pour the mixture into 4 ice pop molds. Freeze for 6 hours before serving.

STORAGE NOTE: You can keep these in the freezer for up to 6 months.

RECIPE TIP: Adding 1 tablespoon of cocoa powder makes this a mocha and boosts the carb count by just 1 gram.

PUMPKIN CHEESECAKE SMOOTHIE

≤15 · GLUTEN-FREE · NUT-FREE · ONE-POT · VEGETARIAN

SERVES 1 · PREP TIME: 10 MINUTES · COOK TIME: NONE

This smoothie is more like a milkshake with the delicious flavors of pumpkin cheesecake. You can omit the cream cheese to make a dairy-free pumpkin pie smoothie. Make sure you use pumpkin purée, which is sugar-free, and not pumpkin pie mix, which has sugar.

2 tablespoons cream cheese, at room temperature

½ cup canned pumpkin purée (not pumpkin pie mix)

1 cup almond milk

1 teaspoon pumpkin pie spice

½ cup crushed ice

PER SERVING Calories: 186; Total Fat: 14g; Saturated Fat: 6g; Sodium: 105mg; Carbohydrates: 14g; Fiber: 5g; Protein: 5g

In a blender, combine all of the ingredients. Blend until smooth.

STORAGE NOTE: This is best when made fresh, although you can refrigerate it overnight. The consistency will be less thick because the ice will melt.

RECIPE TIP: Sprinkle with ¼ cup almond meal for a crust-like topping and an additional 5 grams of carbs and 3 grams of fiber.

CINNAMON SPICED BAKED APPLES

DAIRY-FREE · GLUTEN-FREE · VEGAN

SERVES 4 · PREP TIME: 10 MINUTES · COOK TIME: 15 MINUTES

Whether you eat these apples warm by themselves or let them cool and toss them with some plain yogurt, they are a delicious treat reminiscent of really good apple pie. Use a sweet-tart apple, such as Honeycrisp or Granny Smith. Both of these firm apples hold up well to baking, and the resulting texture and flavor is similar to apple crisp.

2 apples, peeled, cored, and chopped

2 tablespoons pure maple syrup

½ teaspoon cinnamon

½ teaspoon ground ginger

¼ cup chopped pecans

PER SERVING Calories: 122; Total Fat: 5g; Saturated Fat: 0g; Sodium: 2mg; Carbohydrates: 21g; Fiber: 3g; Protein: 1g

1. Preheat the oven to 350°F.

2. In a bowl, mix the apples, syrup, cinnamon, and ginger. Pour the mixture into a 9-inch square baking dish. Sprinkle the pecans over the top.

3. Bake until the apples are tender, about 15 minutes.

STORAGE NOTE: This will keep in the refrigerator for up to 5 days.

RECIPE TIP: Reduce carbs by 4 grams per serving by using only 1 tablespoon of maple syrup whisked with 1 packet of stevia.

BROILED PINEAPPLE

≤15 · DAIRY-FREE · GLUTEN-FREE · NUT-FREE · ONE-POT · VEGAN

SERVES 4 · PREP TIME: 5 MINUTES · COOK TIME: 5 MINUTES

This simple dessert delivers a taste of the tropics. Broiling pineapple brings out its natural sweetness, while toasting the coconut under the broiler adds a deep, caramelized flavor. The sprinkle of sea salt is the perfect contrast for a surprisingly simple and delicious dish.

4 large slices fresh pineapple

2 tablespoons canned coconut milk

2 tablespoons unsweetened shredded coconut

¼ teaspoon sea salt

PER SERVING Calories: 78; Total Fat: 4g; Saturated Fat: 3g; Sodium: 148mg; Carbohydrates: 13g; Fiber: 2g; Protein: 1g

1. Preheat the oven broiler on high.

2. On a rimmed baking sheet, arrange the pineapple in a single layer. Brush lightly with the coconut milk and sprinkle with the coconut.

3. Broil until the pineapple begins to brown, 3 to 5 minutes.

4. Sprinkle with the sea salt.

STORAGE NOTE: This is best fresh and doesn't store well.

RECIPE TIP: While this treat is naturally sweet already, you can whisk up to 1 tablespoon of honey in with the coconut milk before brushing it on the pineapple. This adds 4 grams of carbs per serving but increases caramelization and sweetness.

AVOCADO CHOCOLATE MOUSSE

≤15 · DAIRY-FREE · GLUTEN-FREE · NUT-FREE · ONE-POT · VEGAN

SERVES 4 · PREP TIME: 5 MINUTES · COOK TIME: NONE

If you love chocolate, then using avocados as a mousse base is an inventive way to reduce carbs and increase fiber. It's also really delicious and rich—give it a try! Select avocados that are very soft without being bruised or overripe for best results. Adjust the consistency to your preference by adding more or less coconut milk.

2 avocados, mashed

¼ cup canned coconut milk

2 tablespoons unsweetened cocoa powder

2 tablespoons pure maple syrup

½ teaspoon espresso powder

½ teaspoon vanilla extract

PER SERVING Calories: 203; Total Fat: 17g; Saturated Fat: 7g; Sodium: 11mg; Carbohydrates: 15g; Fiber: 6g; Protein: 2g

1. In a blender, combine all of the ingredients. Blend until smooth.

2. Pour the mixture into 4 small bowls and serve.

STORAGE NOTE: This will keep in the refrigerator for up to 2 days, but you'll want to prevent oxidation of the mousse by pressing plastic wrap directly onto the surface of the mousse so no air reaches it.

RECIPE TIP: Replace the maple syrup with 2 to 3 packets of stevia (choose your sweetness preference—start with less, taste, and add more as needed). This reduces the carbs per serving by 7 grams.

NO-BAKE CHOCOLATE PEANUT BUTTER COOKIES

≤10 · GLUTEN-FREE · VEGETARIAN

MAKES 12 COOKIES · PREP TIME: 10 MINUTES, PLUS 2 HOURS TO CHILL · COOK TIME: NONE

No-bake cookies are quick and easy, and they keep well (see Storage Note). These also travel well and, of course, kids love them. A serving size is 1 cookie, but they offer a little bite of sweetness when you want a treat. Remember to take insulin for snacks, use simple sugars sparingly, and monitor your weight.

¾ cup unsweetened shredded coconut

½ cup peanut butter

2 tablespoons cream cheese, at room temperature

2 tablespoons unsalted butter, melted

2 tablespoons unsweetened cocoa powder

2 tablespoons pure maple syrup

½ teaspoon vanilla extract

PER SERVING (1 cookie) Calories: 143; Total Fat: 12g; Saturated Fat: 7g; Sodium: 13mg; Carbohydrates: 6g; Fiber: 2g; Protein: 4g

1. In a medium bowl, mix all of the ingredients until well combined.

2. Spoon into 12 cookies on a platter lined with parchment paper. Refrigerate to set, about 2 hours.

STORAGE NOTE: Refrigerate in a sealed container for up to 5 days, or freeze for up to 6 months.

RECIPE TIP: Replacing the shredded coconut with ¾ cup of rolled oats increases carbs to about 7 grams per cookie with 2 grams of fiber.

CHOCOLATE ALMOND BUTTER FUDGE

≤10 · DAIRY-FREE · GLUTEN-FREE · VEGAN

MAKES 9 PIECES · PREP TIME: 10 MINUTES, PLUS 3 HOURS TO CHILL · COOK TIME: NONE

When you refrigerate a can of full-fat coconut milk overnight, the liquid settles at the bottom and the coconut cream settles at the top. Spoon off the thickened coconut cream and discard the bottom liquid to get the right texture for this creamy, delicious fudge.

2 ounces unsweetened baking chocolate

½ cup almond butter

1 can full-fat coconut milk, refrigerated overnight, thickened cream only

1 teaspoon vanilla extract

4 (1-gram) packets stevia (or to taste)

PER SERVING (1 piece) Calories: 200; Total Fat: 20g; Saturated Fat: 10g; Sodium: 8mg; Carbohydrates: 6g; Fiber: 2g; Protein: 4g

1. Line a 9-inch square baking pan with parchment paper.

2. In a small saucepan over medium-low heat, heat the chocolate and almond butter, stirring constantly, until both are melted. Cool slightly.

3. In a medium bowl, combine the melted chocolate mixture with the cream from the coconut milk, vanilla, and stevia. Blend until smooth. Taste and adjust sweetness as desired.

4. Pour the mixture into the prepared pan, spreading with a spatula to smooth. Refrigerate for 3 hours. Cut into squares.

STORAGE NOTE: Freeze individual pieces for up to 6 months, or refrigerate for up to 5 days.

RECIPE TIP: Stir in up to ½ cup of chopped almonds to make this dish crunchy—it adds only 1 gram of carbohydrate per serving. Note, however, this is still fudge, so it has calories that can contribute to weight gain. Take insulin, enjoy treats sparingly, keep an eye on body weight and cholesterol levels, and enjoy!

Peri-Peri Sauce (Piri-Piri), page 130

CHAPTER NINE

Sauces and Vinaigrettes

PEA PESTO

It's important to use fresh green peas here, which have the right flavor and texture to make this work. Frozen peas have too high of a water content and will result in a watery pesto. You can also use edamame if you wish.

½ cup fresh green peas

½ cup grated Parmesan cheese

¼ cup fresh basil leaves

¼ cup extra-virgin olive oil

¼ cup pine nuts

2 garlic cloves, minced

¼ teaspoon sea salt

PER SERVING Calories: 248; Total Fat: 23g; Saturated Fat: 4g; Sodium: 338mg; Carbohydrates: 5g; Fiber: 1g; Protein: 7g

In a blender or food processor, combine all of the ingredients. Process until smooth.

STORAGE NOTE: The sauce will store well in the refrigerator for up to 2 days. You can also freeze it in ice cube trays for use in other dishes and sauces. The frozen cubes will last in the freezer for 6 months.

RECIPE TIP: You can try this with edamame without changing the carbohydrate count significantly.

CHIMICHURRI

≤10 · DAIRY-FREE · GLUTEN-FREE · NUT-FREE · ONE-POT · VEGAN

SERVES 4 · PREP TIME: 5 MINUTES · COOK TIME: NONE

Like pesto, chimichurri is a chopped raw green sauce that derives its flavor from herbs and citrus. But while pesto is Italian in origin, chimichurri reflects the flavors popular in Argentina, where it is enjoyed on steak and other meats.

½ cup Italian parsley

¼ cup fresh cilantro, stems removed

¼ cup extra-virgin olive oil

2 tablespoons red wine vinegar

1 garlic clove, minced

Zest of 1 lemon

½ teaspoon sea salt

¼ teaspoon red pepper flakes

PER SERVING Calories: 125; Total Fat: 14g; Saturated Fat: 2g; Sodium: 151mg; Carbohydrates: 1g; Fiber: 0g; Protein: 0g

In a blender or food processor, combine all the ingredients. Process until smooth.

STORAGE NOTE: The sauce will store well in the refrigerator for up to 2 days. You can also freeze it in ice cube trays for use in other dishes and sauces. The frozen cubes will last in the freezer for 6 months.

RECIPE TIP: You can replace the red pepper flakes with half a jalapeño, seeded and chopped. This adds a fresher flavor and changes the heat level. It doesn't significantly change carb counts or fiber.

PERI-PERI SAUCE (PIRI-PIRI)

≤10 · DAIRY-FREE · GLUTEN-FREE · NUT-FREE · VEGAN

SERVES 4 · PREP TIME: 10 MINUTES · COOK TIME: 5 MINUTES

This South African sauce adds tremendous zip to all kinds of foods, including fish and seafood, poultry, meat, and tofu. This is a relatively low-heat version, so feel free to add additional spicy chiles to adjust to your own personal heat preferences.

1 red bell pepper, seeded and chopped

1 red onion, chopped

1 tomato, chopped

4 garlic cloves, minced

1 red chile, seeded and chopped

2 tablespoons extra-virgin olive oil

Juice of 1 lemon

1 tablespoon smoked paprika

1 tablespoon dried oregano

1 teaspoon sea salt

PER SERVING Calories: 99; Total Fat: 7g; Saturated Fat: 1g; Sodium: 296mg; Carbohydrates: 8g; Fiber: 3g; Protein: 1g

1. In a blender or food processor, combine all of the ingredients. Process until smooth.

2. In a small saucepan over medium-high heat, bring the mixture to a simmer, stirring constantly. Reduce heat to medium and simmer for 5 minutes.

STORAGE NOTE: The sauce will store well in the refrigerator for up to 5 days. You can also freeze it in ice cube trays in tablespoon sizes for use in other dishes and sauces. The frozen cubes will last in the freezer for 6 months.

RECIPE TIP: Along with adjusting by using more or spicier chiles, you can also adjust the heat levels upward by adding cayenne or downward by omitting the fresh chile.

REMOULADE

≤10 · DAIRY-FREE · GLUTEN-FREE · NUT-FREE · ONE-POT · VEGETARIAN

SERVES 4 · PREP TIME: 5 MINUTES · COOK TIME: NONE

Remoulade is a creamy, spicy sauce traditionally found in Cajun and Creole cooking, such as in Scallop Po' Boy Lettuce Cups (page 89). However, it also makes a tasty dip for veggies, a yummy burger or sandwich spread, or a dipping sauce for chicken fingers.

¾ cup mayonnaise

2 tablespoons mustard (Creole if you can find it)

1 teaspoon Cajun seasoning

1 teaspoon horseradish

1 teaspoon dill pickle juice

1 garlic clove, minced

½ teaspoon paprika

¼ teaspoon hot pepper sauce (such as Tabasco)

PER SERVING Calories: 180; Total Fat: 15g; Saturated Fat: 2g; Sodium: 410mg; Carbohydrates: 10g; Fiber: 1g; Protein: 1g

In a small bowl, whisk all of the ingredients together until well combined.

STORAGE NOTE: The sauce will store well in the refrigerator for up to 3 days.

RECIPE TIP: If you can't find Creole mustard, any spicy mustard will do. You can adjust heat levels by adding more or less Cajun seasoning, horseradish, and hot pepper sauce.

PUB SAUCE

≤10 · DAIRY-FREE · GLUTEN-FREE · NUT-FREE · ONE-POT

SERVES 4 · PREP TIME: 5 MINUTES · COOK TIME: NONE

This pub sauce is delicious on just about any burger. It also makes a great base for tuna or crab salad, a tasty dip for veggies, or a yummy side dip for chicken fingers or fish sticks.

¼ cup mayonnaise

1 tablespoon pure maple syrup

1 tablespoon reduced-sodium soy sauce

1 tablespoon Worcestershire sauce

1 garlic clove, minced

PER SERVING Calories: 77; Total Fat: 5g; Saturated Fat: 1g; Sodium: 280mg; Carbohydrates: 8g; Fiber: 0g; Protein: 0g

In a small bowl, whisk all the ingredients until well combined.

STORAGE NOTE: The sauce will store well in the refrigerator for up to 3 days.

RECIPE TIP: Add chopped fresh herbs, such as chives, if you wish to pump up the flavor. Adding up to 1 tablespoon of chopped fresh herbs changes the flavor but will not have a significant effect on carbohydrate counts or how you dose insulin.

PEANUT SAUCE

≤10 · DAIRY-FREE · ONE-POT · VEGETARIAN

SERVES 4 · PREP TIME: 5 MINUTES · COOK TIME: NONE

Peanut sauce is great in stir-fries, and it also makes an excellent dip for chicken fingers or topping for seafood or beef. A rasp-style grater is helpful for effectively grating ginger.

¼ cup peanut butter

Juice of 1 lime

1 tablespoon peeled and grated fresh ginger

1 tablespoon honey

1 tablespoon reduced-sodium soy sauce

1 garlic clove, minced

Pinch red pepper flakes

PER SERVING Calories: 118; Total Fat: 8g; Saturated Fat: 2g; Sodium: 137mg; Carbohydrates: 9g; Fiber: 1g; Protein: 4g

In a small bowl, whisk all of the ingredients together until well combined.

STORAGE NOTE: This sauce will store well in the refrigerator for up to 5 days.

RECIPE TIP: You can also use almond butter or cashew butter in place of the peanut butter. Changing the type of nut butter will not change carbohydrate counts significantly. Test blood sugars to determine if you will need to bolus for this sauce. If concerned about body weight, use sauces sparingly.

ASIAN VINAIGRETTE

≤10 · DAIRY-FREE · GLUTEN-FREE · NUT-FREE · ONE-POT · VEGAN

SERVES 2 · PREP TIME: 5 MINUTES · COOK TIME: NONE

This vinaigrette is delicious on salads or slaws. It also makes a nice sauce to spoon over fish or seafood as well as poultry. You can also use it as a poultry, fish, or meat marinade.

¼ cup extra-virgin olive oil

3 tablespoons apple cider vinegar

1 tablespoon peeled and grated fresh ginger

1 tablespoon freshly squeezed lime juice

1 tablespoon chopped fresh cilantro

1 garlic clove, minced

½ teaspoon sriracha

PER SERVING Calories: 252; Total Fat: 27g; Saturated Fat: 4g; Sodium: 3mg; Carbohydrates: 2g; Fiber: <1g; Protein: 0g

In a small bowl, whisk all of the ingredients together until well combined.

STORAGE NOTE: This sauce will store well in the refrigerator for up to 5 days. Whisk before using.

RECIPE TIP: Adjust the sriracha quantity to adjust spiciness. You can also add up to ½ teaspoon of Chinese hot mustard, which will raise heat levels and help emulsify the dressing. If you add Chinese hot mustard, this will no longer be gluten-free. However, it won't affect carb levels much.

ITALIAN/GREEK VINAIGRETTE

≤10 · DAIRY-FREE · GLUTEN-FREE · NUT-FREE · ONE-POT · VEGAN

SERVES 4 · PREP TIME: 5MINUTES · COOK TIME: NONE

This basic recipe allows you to make two different vinaigrettes: Italian and Greek. Carb counts are about the same for each, as is the process for making them. The only difference is in the ingredients.

ITALIAN

¼ cup extra-virgin olive oil

2 tablespoons red wine vinegar

1 tablespoon minced shallot

2 teaspoons Italian seasoning

1 garlic clove, finely minced

1 teaspoon Dijon mustard

¼ teaspoon sea salt

⅛ teaspoon freshly ground black pepper

GREEK

¼ cup extra virgin olive oil

1 tablespoon red wine vinegar

1 tablespoon freshly squeezed lemon juice

3 garlic cloves, minced

1 teaspoon dried oregano

1 teaspoon dried marjoram

½ teaspoon lemon zest

¼ teaspoon sea salt

In a small bowl, whisk all of the ingredients together until well combined.

STORAGE NOTE: Both vinaigrettes will store well in the refrigerator for up to 5 days. Whisk before using.

RECIPE TIP: Add heat to either dressing with a pinch of red pepper flakes.

PER SERVING Calories: 127; Total Fat: 14g; Saturated Fat: 2g; Sodium: 74mg; Carbohydrates: 1g; Fiber: <1g; Protein: 0g

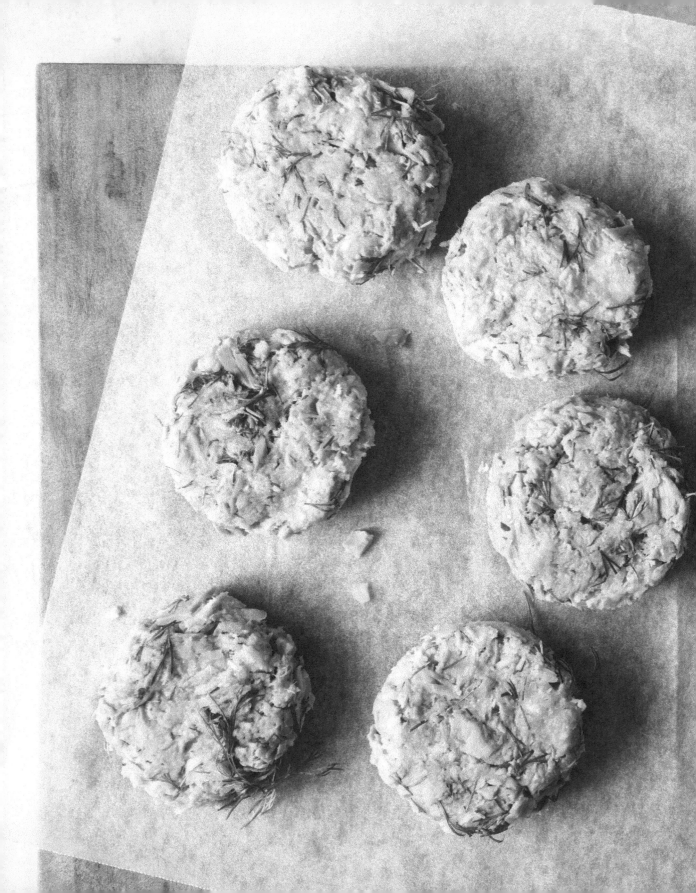

APPENDIX A
How Many Calories Do You Need?

Type 1 diabetes typically does not indicate the need for calorie counting. However, understanding your calorie (energy) requirements will provide a starting point for you to figure out your daily estimated carbohydrate requirements. First, find out how many calories you need; next, look at Appendix B to see what percentage of calories may come from carbohydrates. Knowing this information may help you achieve a balanced diet, control weight, and stabilize blood sugar levels.

Sedentary means a lifestyle that includes only the physical activity of independent living.

Moderately Active means a lifestyle that includes physical activity equivalent to walking 1.5 to 3 miles per day at 3 to 4 miles per hour, in addition to the activities of independent living.

Active means a lifestyle that includes physical activity equivalent to walking more than 3 miles per day at 3 to 4 miles per hour, in addition to the activities of independent living.

Estimates for females do not include women who are pregnant or breastfeeding.

Source: Institute of Medicine. Dietary Reference Intakes for Energy, Carbohydrate, Fiber, Fat, Fatty Acids, Cholesterol, Protein, and Amino Acids. *Washington, DC: National Academies Press, 2002.*

| | MALES | | | FEMALES | | |
| | Activity Level | | | Activity Level | | |
Age	Sedentary*	Mod. Active*	Active	Sedentary*	Mod. Active*	Active
2	1000	1000	1000	1000	1000	1000
3	1000	1400	1400	1000	1200	1400
4	1200	1400	1600	1200	1400	1400
5	1200	1400	1600	1200	1400	1600
6	1400	1600	1800	1200	1400	1600
7	1400	1600	1800	1200	1600	1800
8	1400	1600	2000	1400	1600	1800

Age	MALES			FEMALES		
	Activity Level			Activity Level		
	Sedentary*	Mod. Active*	Active	Sedentary*	Mod. Active*	Active
9	1600	1800	2000	1400	1600	1800
10	1600	1800	2200	1400	1800	2000
11	1800	2000	2200	1600	1800	2000
12	1800	2200	2400	1600	2000	2200
13	2000	2200	2600	1600	2000	2200
14	2000	2400	2800	1800	2000	2400
15	2200	2600	3000	1800	2000	2400
16	2400	2800	3200	1800	2000	2400
17	2400	2800	3200	1800	2000	2400
18	2400	2800	3200	1800	2000	2400
19–20	2600	2800	3000	2000	2200	2400
21–25	2400	2800	3000	2000	2200	2400
26–30	2400	2600	3000	1800	2000	2400
31–35	2400	2600	3000	1800	2000	2200
36–40	2400	2600	2800	1800	2000	2200
41–45	2200	2600	2800	1800	2000	2200
46–50	2200	2400	2800	1800	2000	2200
51–55	2200	2400	2800	1600	1800	2200
56-60	2200	2400	2600	1600	1800	2200
61–65	2000	2400	2600	1600	1800	2000
66–70	2000	2200	2600	1600	1800	2000
71–75	2000	2200	2600	1600	1800	2000
76 and up	2000	2200	2400	1600	1800	2000

How Many Carbohydrates Do You Need?

The recommended amount of carbs is individualized and often based on energy requirements. Carb grams are calculated as a percentage of your total calories.* The National Academy of Medicine recommends no fewer than 130 grams of carbs daily.

CALORIES	CARBOHYDRATE GRAMS				
	35%	40%	45%	50%	55%
1000	87	100	112	125	137
1100	96	110	123	137	151
1200	105	120	135	150	165
1300	113	130	146	162	178
1400	122	140	157	175	192
1500	131	150	168	187	206
1600	140	160	180	200	220
1700	148	170	191	212	233
1800	157	180	202	225	247
1900	166	190	213	237	261
2000	175	200	225	250	275
2100	183	210	236	262	288
2200	192	220	247	275	302
2300	201	230	258	287	316
2400	210	240	270	300	330
2500	218	250	281	312	343
2600	227	260	292	325	357
2700	236	270	303	337	371
2800	245	280	315	350	385
2900	253	290	326	362	398
3000	262	300	337	375	412

*Carbohydrates contain 4 calories per gram

APPENDIX C
Carbohydrate Counts for Diverse Menus

Estimating carbohydrate counts at mealtime is easier if you understand the carbohydrate values of foods that are consistent with your individual food preferences, culture, and lifestyle. Take a look at some of the common foods that you may use while preparing meals, dining out, or traveling. Additional information on carbohydrate counting is available from the many resource applications that are listed on page 144.

FOOD TYPE	SERVING SIZE	CARB GRAMS	CALORIES
ASIAN			
Amaranth (Chinese spinach)	1 cup, cooked	6	28
Bamboo shoots	½ cup, canned	2	13
Carambola/star fruit	1 (3⅝ inches long)	14	60
Cellophane noodles	½ cup, cooked	16	67
Kohlrabi	1 cup, boiled	11	48
Lychee	10, raw	15	63
Moon cake	1½ ounces	24	169
Mung beans	½ cup, cooked	16	67
Persimmon	½ fruit	15	59
Rice	1 cup, cooked	44	199
Rice noodles	½ cup, cooked	23	99
Taro	½ cup, cooked	22	94
Udon noodles	1 cup, cooked	43	210
CAJUN/CREOLE			
Alligator	1 ounce	0	42
Cracklins	¼ cup	0	131
Cushaw squash	½ cup	9	41
Frog legs	1½ ounces, steamed	0	45
Kumquats	5	15	60

FOOD TYPE	SERVING SIZE	CARB GRAMS	CALORIES
Lamb	1 ounce	0	83
Passion fruit/maypops	3	12	52
Pumpkin	½ cup	5	20
Salt pork	½ cubic inch	0	45
Tripe	2 ounces, cooked	0	57
FILIPINO			
Beef shank	1 ounce	0	57
Bihon/rice sticks	¾ cup	18	91
Bitter melon	1 cup, raw	3	16
Cassava tuber	½ cup	39	165
Chicken gizzard/balunbalunan	1 ounce	0	43
Guava	1 cup	24	112
Jicama	1 cup	11	49
Kalabasa/banana squash	½ cup	6	24
Mung bean noodles/sotanghon	¾ cup	18	73
Oysters/talaba	1 medium	2	41
INDIAN			
Aloo gobi (potato and cauliflower)	1 cup	15	80
Chapati/roti	6-inch diameter	15	80
Chicken curry	1¼ cups	15	125
Dosa	10-inch diameter	15	80
Idli	1½ ounces	15	80
Mung dal	½ cup, cooked	15	125
Paneer	1 ounce	6	90
Seetaphal (custard apple)	1 medium	15	60
Upma	½ cup	15	80
ITALIAN			
Burrata	1 ounce	1	80
Italian bread crumbs	¼ cup	23	130
Mozzarella cheese	1 ounce	1	120
Olive oil	1 tablespoon	0	120
Parmesan cheese	1 ounce, grated	1	122
Polenta	⅓ cup, cooked	15	80
Shrimp	4 ounces	0	120
Spaghetti/pasta	1 cup, cooked	41	210

FOOD TYPE	SERVING SIZE	CARB GRAMS	CALORIES
Steamed clams	24	4	120
Stewed tomato	½ cup	8	80
Veal chop	3 ounces, cooked	0	180
JEWISH			
Bialy/bagel	2 ounces	30	160
Bulgur	½ cup, cooked	17	76
Challah	1 ounce	15	80
Chicken, white meat	1 ounce, cooked	0	35
Flanken	1 ounce, cooked	0	57
Herring	1 ounce	0	61
Kasha	½ cup, cooked	20	91
Lox	1 ounce	0	33
Matzo balls	3 small	17	134
Pastrami	1 ounce	0	99
MEXICAN			
Avocado	⅛ medium	2	40
Beans/frijoles	⅓ cup	14	80
Cassava	1 cup	78	328
Chayote	1 cup, boiled	8	40
Chicken leg	3 ounces	0	156
Chorizo	1 ounce	0	132
Crayfish	3 ounces	0	70
Mango	½ small	17	68
Sopadilla	3 ounces	19	71
Tortilla, corn	7½-inch diameter	13	70
VEGAN			
Black beans	½ cup, cooked	20	113
Cashew butter	1 tablespoon	4	94
Edamame	½ cup, frozen	9	100
Flaxseed	1 tablespoon, ground	2	30
Hemp	3 tablespoons	2.6	166
Quinoa	1 cup, cooked	39	223
Seaweed (laver)	3 sheets	<1	3
Soy milk	1 cup	14	140
Soy nut butter	2 tablespoons	10	190
Tempeh	3 ounces, cooked	8	167

Measurement Conversions

VOLUME EQUIVALENTS (LIQUID)

U.S. STANDARD	U.S. STANDARD (ounces)	METRIC (approximate)
2 tablespoons	1 fl. oz.	30 mL
¼ cup	2 fl. oz.	60 mL
½ cup	4 fl. oz.	120 mL
1 cup	8 fl. oz.	240 mL
1½ cups	12 fl. oz.	355 mL
2 cups or 1 pint	16 fl. oz.	475 mL
4 cups or 1 quart	32 fl. oz.	1 L
1 gallon	128 fl. oz.	4 L

OVEN TEMPERATURES

FAHRENHEIT	CELSIUS (approximate)
250°F	120°C
300°F	150°C
325°F	165°C
350°F	180°C
375°F	190°C
400°F	200°C
425°F	220°C
450°F	230°C

VOLUME EQUIVALENTS (DRY)

U.S. STANDARD	METRIC (approximate)
⅛ teaspoon	0.5 mL
¼ teaspoon	1 mL
½ teaspoon	2 mL
¾ teaspoon	4 mL
1 teaspoon	5 mL
1 tablespoon	15 mL
¼ cup	59 mL
⅓ cup	79 mL
½ cup	118 mL
⅔ cup	156 mL
¾ cup	177 mL
1 cup	235 mL
2 cups or 1 pint	475 mL
3 cups	700 mL
4 cups or 1 quart	1 L

WEIGHT EQUIVALENTS

U.S. STANDARD	METRIC (approximate)
½ ounce	15 g
1 ounce	30 g
2 ounces	60 g
4 ounces	115 g
8 ounces	225 g
12 ounces	340 g
16 ounces or 1 pound	455 g

Resources for Diabetes Education

CALCULATION TOOLS

CALORIE KING
www.calorieking.com
A food database providing accurate information about the nutritional value of the foods we eat each day. Includes fast food restaurants and supermarket brands.

CARB AND CALS
www.carbsandcals.com
Visual learners who are carbohydrate counting will love the extensive photo database available for iPhone and Android devices. Meals and foods have been nutritionally analyzed. The app allows you to compare what you are eating to the photos in the database. You can also add custom foods. The app has the ability to calculate total carbohydrates and brings attention to portion sizes at meals.

MY FITNESS PAL
www.myfitnesspal.com/recipe/calculator
Recipe nutrition calculator and fitness tracker.

UNITED STATES DEPARTMENT OF AGRICULTURE
USDA FOOD COMPOSITION DATABASE
https://ndb.nal.usda.gov/ndb/search/list
Extensive database of foods in all categories that enable you to analyze not only the carbohydrates but also the vitamins and minerals in the food that you eat.

UNIVERSITY OF SYDNEY GLYCEMIC INDEX
www.glycemicindex.com/foodSearch.php
Complete listing of foods and their glycemic index.

SMARTPHONE CARB-COUNTING APPS

Calorie King
Carbs and Cals
Glucose Buddy Diabetes
My Fitness Pal
MyNetDiary's Diabetes and Diet Tracker

ORGANIZATIONS

AMERICAN ASSOCIATION OF DIABETES EDUCATORS
DiabetesEducator.org
This site is very useful for those looking for a nationally recognized diabetes education program or a certified diabetes educator. You will also find extensive, reliable information that has been reviewed by certified diabetes educators. Provides an excellent resource app at danaapps.org.

AMERICAN DIABETES ASSOCIATION
Diabetes.org
The ADA is a leading organization that will keep you informed about current research and development in all areas of diabetes. Membership entitles you to receive its lifestyle magazine, *Diabetes Forecast*, which is a helpful resource for a wide range of diabetes-related topics, including nutrition, exercise, medication, and technology.

BEYOND TYPE 1
beyondtype1.org
Founded in 2015, by Nick Jonas, Juliet Raubigny, Sarah Lucas and Sam Talbot. These celebrities, all living with type 1, joined together to educate the global community about managing blood sugars. The organization's website is creative and features extensive information and resources; be sure to look at information on travel, adventures, holidays, and clinical trials.

CHILDREN WITH DIABETES
ChildrenWithDiabetes.org
A favorite diabetes resource for children, young adults, parents, and caregivers. This user-friendly website provides age-appropriate educational materials, including ideas about navigating school, scholarships, camp, sports, exercise, and nutrition. Be sure to check out Quilts for Life, art projects illustrated by children with diabetes.

DIABETIC CONNECT
DiabeticConnect.com

Encourages conversations and discussions with other members of the diabetes community. This social network discusses a wide range of topics ranging from recipes to insulin pumps. An "Ask the Expert" section is divided into categories with easy-to-understand information on many current topics.

DIABETES SISTERS
DiabetesSisters.org

Excellent and empowering support and advocacy website for women living with diabetes. Extensive resources that encourage women to communicate with one another online or via local meetups.

DIATRIBE
Diatribe.org

Actionable tips and cutting-edge ideas to help individuals with diabetes. Many links to information on pump therapy, medications, sensors, insurance, and support systems. Excellent list of blogs and forums.

ETHNOMED
http://ethnomed.org/patient-education/diabetes

Thank goodness for this website. It supplies culturally sensitive diabetes education materials. Video and written materials are available in different languages.

INTERNATIONAL DIABETES FEDERATION
IDF.org

More than 160 countries and 230 national diabetes associations collaborate to help the world understand more about diabetes through IDF. This global organization's initiatives include IDF Diabetes Atlas, World Diabetes Day, and Congress for Life. Resources for diabetes education are available in different languages through this site.

JDRF
JDRF.org

Previously called the Juvenile Diabetes Research Foundation, this organization has local chapters geared toward bringing families together for walks, cycling, seminars, and support groups. Provides free "Bags of Hope" for those initially diagnosed. Donations fund diabetes research aimed at curing diabetes.

References

American Diabetes Association. "Standards of Medical Care in Diabetes–2018." *Diabetes Care* 41, suppl. 1 (January 2018): S1–S2. doi.org/10.2337/dc18-Sint01.

American Dietetic Association and American Diabetes Association. *Ethnic and Regional Food Practices–A Series.* Chicago: Academy of Nutrition and Dietetics, 1989–99.

Balk, Ethan M., Athina Tatsioni, Alice H. Lichtenstein, Joseph Lau, and Anastassios G. Pittas. "The Effect of Chromium Supplementation on Glucose Metabolism and Lipids." *Diabetes Care* 30, no. 8 (August 2007): 2154–63. Accessed June 1, 2018. https://doi.org/10.2337/dc06-0996.

Bell, Kirstine, Alan Barclay, Peter Petocz, Stephen Colagiuri, and Jennie Brand-Mille. "Efficacy of Carbohydrate Counting in Type 1 Diabetes: A Systematic Review and Meta-Analysis." *The Lancet Diabetes & Endocrinology* 2, no. 2 (February 2014): 133–40. doi.org/10.1016/S2213-8587(13)70144-X.

Benjamin, Evan. "Self-Monitoring of Blood Glucose: The Basics." *Clinical Diabetes* 20, no. 1 (January 2002): 45–47. https://doi.org/10.2337/diaclin.20.1.45.

Brown-Riggs, Constance. "Low-Carb Diets & Diabetes." *Today's Dietitian* 18, no. 8 (August 2016): 24. http://www.todaysdietitian.com/newarchives/0816p24.shtml.

Calorie King Guide. https://www.calorieking.com. Accessed July 18, 2018.

Chandran, Manju, and Steve Edelman. "Have Insulin, Will Fly: Diabetes Management During Air Travel and Time Zone Adjustment Strategies" *Clinical Diabetes* 21, no. 2 (2003): 82–85. https://doi.org/10.2337/diaclin.21.2.82.

De Oliveira, Vanessa Rabello Lovisi Sales, and Caroline Pereira Domingueti. "Association of Vitamin D Deficiency and Type 1 Diabetes Mellitus: A Systematic Review and Meta-Anaylsis." *International Journal of Diabetes in Developing Countries* (2018). https://doi.org/10.1007/s13410-018-0607-4.

Edwards, Alison. "An Introduction to Carbohydrate Counting in Type 1 Diabetes." *Journal of Diabetes Nursing* 19, no. 2 (2015): 73–77.

Feinman, Richard D., Wendy K. Pogozelski, Arne Astrup, Richard K. Bernstein, Eugene J. Fine, Eric C. Westman, Anthony Accurso, et al. "Dietary Carbohydrate Restriction as the First Approach in Diabetes Management: Critical Review and Evidence Base." *Nutrition* 31, no. 1 (2015): 1–13. doi.org/10.1016/j.nut.2014.06.011

Food and Agriculture Organization of the United Nations. "International Network of Food Data Systems (INFOODS)." Accessed July 21, 2018. http://www.fao.org/infoods/infoods /tables-and-databases/en/.

Foster-Powell, Kaye, Susanna H. A. Holt, and Janette C. Brand-Miller. "International Table of Glycemic Index and Glycemic Load Values: 2002." *American Journal of Clinical Nutrition* 76, no. 1, (July 1, 2002): 5–56. https://doi.org/10.1093/ajcn/76.1.5.

Goff, Louise PhD, RF; Dyson, Pamela PhD, RD, British Dietetic Association. Advanced Nutrition and Dietetics In Diabetes Nutrition Management of Glycaemia in Type 1 Diabetes Care. Wiley Online Books (October 23, 2015): 67–73. www.wiley.com/en-us /Advanced+Nutrition+and+Dietetics+in+Diabetes-p-9780470670927

Hamza, Nasir, and Narasimhan, Sumana. "Type 1 Diabetes: The Need for Culture-Appropriate Information on Carbohydrate Counting." *The Lancet Diabetes-Endocrinology* 4 (October 2016): 812. https://doi.org/10.1016/S2213-8587(16)30101-2.

Heaton, Kenneth, Samuel Marcus, Pauline Emmett, and Colin Bolton. "Particle Size of Wheat, Maize and Oat Test Meals: Effect on Plasma Glucose and Insulin Responses and on the Rate of Starch Digestion in Vitro." *American Journal of Clinical Nutrition* 47, no. 4 (May 1988): 675–682. https://doi.org/10.1093/ajcn/47.4.675.

Kulkarni, Karmeen. "Carbohydrate Counting: A Practical Meal Planning Option for People with Diabetes." *Clinical Diabetes* 23, no. 3 (July 2005): 120–22. https://doi.org/10.2337/diaclin.23.3.120.

Lilly Diabetes. *My Carbohydrate Guide.* Accessed July 31, 2018. http://www.lillydiabetes.com /_assets/pdf/ld90766_carbguide.pdf.

Lind, Marcus, William Polonsky, Irl Hirsch, Tim Heise, Jan Bolinder, Sofia Dalqvist, Erik Schwarz, et al. "Continuous Glucose Monitoring vs Conventional Therapy for Glycemic Control in Adults with Type 1, Treatment with Multiple Daily Injections, The GOLD Randomized Clinical Trial." *JAMA* 317, no. 4 (2017): 379–87. Accessed July 27, 2018. https://jamanetwork.com/journals /jama/fullarticle/2598771.

Martin, Theresa, and R. Keith Campbell. "Vitamin D and Diabetes." *Diabetes Spectrum* 24, no. 2 (May 2011): 113–18. https://doi.org/10.2337/diaspect.24.2.113.

National Institutes of Health. (May 2015). https://www.bones.nih.gov/health-info/bone /bone-health/nutrition/calcium-and-vitamin-d-important-every-age.

Office of Disease Prevention and Health Promotion. "2015–2020 Dietary Guidelines for Americans." https://health.gov/dietaryguidelines/2015/guidelines/.

Palinski-Wade, Erin. "Changes Are Coming to the New Nutrition Facts Label." *Diabetes Forecast* (March 2018). http://www.diabetesforecast.org/2018/02-mar-apr/changes-are-coming-to -the.html.

Riddell, Michael C., Ian W. Gallen, Carmel E. Smart, Craig E. Taplin, Peter Adolfsson, Alistair N. Lumb, Aaron Kowalski, et al. "Exercise Management and Type 1 Diabetes: A Consensus

Statement." *The Lancet Diabetes and Endocrinology* 5, no. 5: 377–90. Accessed June 1, 2018. https://doi.org/10.1016/S2213-8587(17)30014-1.

Salis, Sheryl. "A Quick Guide to Carbohydrate Counting for Insulin Pump Users." Accessed July 29, 2018. https://endokids.files.wordpress.com/2016/11/carbohydrate-counting1.pdf.

Scheiner, Gary. "Counting Carbohydrates Like a Pro." *Diabetes Self-Management*. Last modified January 13, 2017. https://www.diabetesselfmanagement.com/nutrition-exercise /meal-planning/counting-carbohydrates-like-a-pro/.

Sunberg, Frida, Kathrine Barnard, Allison Cato, Carine de Beaufort, Linda A. DiMeglio, Greg Dooley, Tamara Hershey, et al. "Managing Diabetes in Preschool Children." *Pediatric Diabetes* (2017): 1–19. https://doi.org/10.1111/pedi.12554.

U.S. Department of Agriculture, National Institute of Health: Office of Dietary Supplements. "Chromium Dietary Supplement Fact Sheet." March 2, 2018. https://ods.od.nih.gov/factsheets /Chromium-HealthProfessional/.

U.S. Department of Agriculture. "USDA Food Composition Databases." http://ndb.nal.usda.gov /ndb/search/list.

U.S. Food and Drug Administration. "A Food Labeling Guide. Guidance for Industry." Accessed July 27, 2018. https://www.fda.gov/downloads/Food/GuidanceRegulation/GuidanceDocuments RegulatoryInformation/UCM265446.pdf.

U.S. Food and Drug Administration. "Guidance for Industry: Food Labeling Guide." January 2013. http://www.fda.gov/FoodLabelingGuide.

Wagle, Ashwini. "Carbohydrate Counting for Traditional South Asian Foods." Accessed July 31, 2018. http://www.sjsu.edu/people/ashwini.wagle/Southasians/Carbohydrate%20Counting%20 Tool%20for%20South%20Asians%204th%20Version.pdf.

Walsh, John, and Ruth Roberts. *Pumping Insulin: Everything for Success on an Insulin Pump and CGM*, 6th ed. San Diego, CA: Torrey Pines Press, 2015.

Zhukouskay, Volha, Alla Shepelkevich, and Iacopo Chiodini. "Bone Health in Type 1 Diabetes: Where We Are Now and How Should We Proceed?" *Advances in Endocrinology* 2014, Article ID 982129: 1–12. http://dx.doi.org/10.1155/2014/982129.

Recipe Index

Index

Acknowledgments

Thank you, Callisto Media: my editor, Meg Ilasco; Elizabeth Castoria; Karen Frazier; Erum Khan; Patty Consolazio; and Robin Donovan. With thanks to Martha McKittrick, RDN, CDE; Zoltan Antal, MD; Alexis Feuer, MD; Marisa Censani, MD; Jane Seley, DNP, MPH, CDE; Athena Philis-Tsimikas, MD, Richard Mahler, MD; Richard Weil, MEd, CDE; and Jason Baker, MD. You have all taught me so much about diabetes and patient care. Special appreciation to everyone at the Scripps Whittier Diabetes Institute, New York Presbyterian Hospital, and Weill Cornell Medicine; your passion and dedication to health care is state-of-the-art. Thank you, Keith and Larry, for always challenging me; Ronnie, Howard, and Fern, for always thinking differently; Brian, my son, for inspiring me in the kitchen; Mom, who never stops believing in me; and my husband, Michael, for eating with me all over the world, always being supportive, and helping me chase my dreams.

About the Author

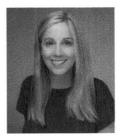

Laurie Block, MS, RDN, CDE, is a nutritionist/registered dietitian and certified diabetes educator practicing in New York City and San Diego, California. Laurie specializes in diabetes with particular interest in type 1. She has consulted with diabetes programs throughout the United States and has lectured on behalf of the Juvenile Diabetes Research Foundation. She is a strong advocate of food and nutrition in the prevention of disease and uses evidence-based recommendations when counseling diverse populations of all age-groups. Creative and collaborative in her approach, Laurie combines a traditional treatment method with modern technology to educate individuals about the ever-changing science of nutrition and how it relates to diabetes management.

Printed in the USA
CPSIA information can be obtained
at www.ICGtesting.com
JSHW040214010424
59884JS00004B/16

9 781641 522335